FEMINIST PERSPECTIVES SERIES

Series Editors:

Professor Pamela Abbott, University of Teesside
Professor Claire Wallace, University of Derby and Institute for
Advanced Studies, Vienna

Published Titles:

Feminist perspectives on the body
Barbara Brook

Feminist perspectives on politics
Chris Corrin

Feminist perspectives on language
Margaret Gibbon

Feminist perspectives on ethics
Elizabeth Porter

Forthcoming Titles:

Feminist perspectives on postcolonialism
Maryanne Dever and Denise Cuthbert

Feminist perspectives on domestic violence
Laura Goldsack and Jill Radford

Feminist perspectives on environment and society
Beate Littig and Barbara Hegenbart

FEMINIST PERSPECTIVES SERIES

Feminist Perspectives on Disability

Barbara Fawcett

An imprint of **Pearson Education**

Harlow, England · London · New York · Reading, Massachusetts · San Francisco
Toronto · Don Mills, Ontario · Sydney · Tokyo · Singapore · Hong Kong · Seoul
Taipei · Cape Town · Madrid · Mexico City · Amsterdam · Munich · Paris · Milan

Pearson Education Limited
Edinburgh Gate
Harlow
Essex CM20 2JE
England
and Associated Companies throughout the world

Visit us on the World Wide Web at:
http://www.pearsoneduc.com

First published 2000

© Pearson Education Limited 2000

The right of Barbara Fawcett to be identified
as author of this Work has been asserted by
her in accordance with the Copyright,
Designs and Patents Act 1988.

ISBN 0 582 36941 X

British Library Cataloguing-in-Publication Data
A catalogue record for this book is available from the British Library

Library of Congress Cataloging-in-Publication Data
A catalog record for this book is available from the Library of Congress

Typeset by 35 in 10/12pt New Baskerville
Produced by Pearson Education Asia Pte Ltd.
Printed in Singapore

Contents

Acknowledgements

It is at this point that I would like to express my deepest thanks to Maurice, Katie and Sophie for all the help they have given me with this book. It would not have been possible without them.

I would also like to fully acknowledge the academic support provided by Maurice Hanlon, Professor Jeff Hearn and Brid Featherstone.

Chapter 1

Setting the scene

> *Now we must recognise differences among [disabled people] who are our equals, neither inferior nor superior, and devise ways to use each others' difference to enrich our visions and our joint struggles.*
>
> (Audre Lorde 1984: 122; 'disabled people' has been substituted for 'women')

Chapter outline

An overview of key issues in terms of writing about disability:

- who should write about disability?
- feminism(s) as opposed to feminism
- 'disabled people' and 'women' as undifferentiated unitary groupings
- the place of experience
- issues about appropriation
- the structure of the book overall

Introduction

Disability and writing about disability are currently regarded as contentious areas. The formulation of the social model of disability has resulted in searing attacks on previously accepted ways of viewing disability and also upon non-disabled authors and writers 'colonising' the field and producing material of little benefit to disabled people (Oliver 1996). In turn, although there are notable exceptions, issues of gender are only just starting to feature strongly in writings which emphasise the social model of disability. In an introduction to a book focusing on feminist perspectives of disability, these are areas which require consideration.

In this chapter, as a means of setting the scene, various feminist perspectives associated with liberal feminism, radical feminism, socialist feminism, black feminism and ecofeminism, will be reviewed. The difficulties associated with viewing 'disabled people' and women as homogeneous, unified groupings rather than as very different and diverse associations will also be explored. Additionally, issues related to writing about 'disability' will be appraised and concerns such as those voiced by Oliver (1996) examined.

The language used in relation to 'disability' will be critically reviewed throughout this book. However, it is useful to point out at this early stage that with regard to general definitions of 'disability' and 'impairment', the formulations devised by the Union of Physically Impaired Against Segregation (UPIAS) will be adhered to. These definitions are explored in more detail in Chapter 2, but it is pertinent to outline at this point, that 'impairment' is defined as 'lacking part of or all of a limb or having a defective limb, organ or mechanism of the body' and 'disability' is defined as 'the disadvantage or restriction of activity caused by a contemporary social organisation which takes no or little account of people who have mainstream impairments and thus excludes them from participation in the mainstream of social activities' (UPIAS 1976, cited in Oliver 1996: 22).

Feminist perspectives

Within feminist movements, there is now an acknowledgement that there are feminisms as opposed to feminism. Key distinctions can be made between 'liberal' feminism and 'radical' feminism. Additional feminisms can be identified as socialist feminism, black feminism and ecofeminism. Jary and Jary (1991), drawing from Palmer (1989), also list academic feminism, cultural feminism (which is also associated with radical feminism), lesbian feminism, psychoanalytic feminism and political lesbianism. A brief outline is given below of the first five feminisms cited and it has to be borne in mind that within these feminisms there are also many points of overlap and multiple variations.

Liberal feminism is wide-ranging, but generally there can be seen to be a focus on a critique of socialisation processes and the creation of sex role stereotypes. Attention is drawn particularly to the unequal ways in which women, as compared to men, have been treated in educational and employment spheres and the manner in which occupations regarded as 'female' have been devalued. Emphasis is placed on issues of equality, on changing socialisation processes, on re-education and upon legislative measures to overcome discrimination. Sexual difference and a focus on women's particular needs and characteristics are not highlighted and equality is seen as obtainable. As Prince (1993) points out, there is an appeal to the inherent rationality of individuals and a belief that practices, such as positive discrimination, anti-sexist education and the identification of positive female role models, should alter perceptions and result in a genuine equality of opportunities and experiences. There can be seen to be many similarities here with exponents of the social model of disability with its insistence on autonomy, control and enforceable equal rights legislation.

Radical feminism is also wide-ranging. However, in contrast to liberal feminism, there is a strong critique of patriarchy. Women's differences from men are revalued and positively highlighted and power imbalances are emphasised. Differential treatment for women and men is seen to result from the ways in which formal social structures (education, marriage, etc.) reinforce and reproduce women's negative positioning. Rather than re-education being emphasised, there is a focus on challenging masculinist systems which are presented as being rational, objective and neutral. Feminist standpoint theory can be seen to have links with this perspective, as can orientations developed by writers such as Irigaray (1993) which celebrate difference and separatism by focusing on cultural and historical factors, rather than on biological factors.

Socialist feminism has sought to incorporate a class analysis within a liberatory perspective. Women's class position within capitalism and the subordinate positioning of women within the family are seen as the basis for challenge. Economic exploitation and sexual oppression are regarded as key focal points, but there are tensions in that economic exploitation relates to class position and will not apply to all women, whilst sexual oppression arguably will. As Jackson (1993) points out, Marxism has been found by many to be an unwieldy and inappropriate tool for exploring gender divisions. This has resulted in many feminists focusing on the cultural construction of masculinity and femininity as a means of overcoming women's oppression.

Ecofeminism links campaigns to end oppression against women with campaigns to end the exploitation of the ecosystem, whilst black feminism(s) is concerned with addressing racism both within and beyond women's movements and highlighting and countering the particular oppressions that face black women. Stanlie M. James asserts that black feminism(s) is about both theorising and taking 'a proactive/reactive stance of pragmatic activism which addresses those issues deemed deleterious to the well-being of black women' (James 1993: 2). Black feminism posed a key challenge to the assumed universality of the feminist movement in the 1970s and can be seen to have paved the way for explorations of difference and diversity. Similar challenges can be seen to be emerging in relation to the 'universalism' of disabled people's movements, based on the social model of disability, by calls for the inclusion of issues related to gender, 'race', impairment, ethnicity and age.

The critique of knowledge frameworks, seen to be dominated by white male eurocentric perspectives, has been a key feature of all feminisms. The various feminisms have therefore sought alternative ways of generating knowledge. Harding (1986, 1990) maintains that three distinct strands can be identified. These are feminist empiricism which seeks to identify and remove sexist and androcentric bias by stricter adherence to existing methodological scientific enquiry; feminist standpoint, which by exploring women's lives from feminist perspectives and by taking full account of experiences of oppression claims to produce a less distorted and more realistic form of knowledge than previously; and feminist postmodernism. Harding does not regard these strands as distinct and separate and there are many points of overlap. Although Harding uses arguments derived from postmodern feminist perspectives to critique feminist standpoint and feminist empiricism, she appears reluctant to embrace postmodern feminist perspectives because of the implications for the deconstruction of gender.[1] She also argues that in relation to political action, a standpoint approach has to have a place. In relation to how these approaches have been linked to feminism(s), some forms of feminist empiricism have been associated with liberal feminism and there are links between feminist standpoint and radical feminism, although reformulations of standpoint epistemology (e.g. Hartsock 1996), discussed further in Chapter 3, have points of comparison with postmodern feminism(s).

Within disability rights movements based on the social model of disability, emphasis is placed both on the challenging of able-bodied knowledge claims and on personal experiences of disablism. However, there is a clear focus on the full integration of disabled people into society on the basis of rights-based citizenship entitlements, rather than in relation to separatist claims. Criticism of the

social model of disability has tended to result in calls for the further development of the model, for greater theorisation, and for
issues of gender, impairment, difference and diversity to be taken
into account, rather than for different models or conceptualisations
to be formulated. Many writers have contributed (e.g. French 1993;
Morris 1993a, 1996a; Crow 1996; Shakespeare 1996; Wendell 1996;
Pinder 1996, 1997; Johnston 1997; Shakespeare and Watson 1997)
and their suggestions will be reviewed in the context of the discussion relating to how feminism(s) can be used both as a point of
comparison and as a critical tool with regard to the social model
of disability and disability rights movements. These areas are discussed in Chapter 3.

Undifferentiated unitary groupings

This area is considered in greater detail in Chapter 3, but it is
important to emphasise here the difficulties associated with viewing
'women' or 'disabled people' as comprising undifferentiated unitary groupings. Diverse organisations such as government agencies,
social services departments, health trusts, exponents of disability
rights campaigns and feminist organisations in the early 1970s, all
use or have used such broad-brush categorisation processes. With
regard to feminism in the 1970s, as Fawcett and Featherstone
(1994a) outline, there was a strong commitment to resisting the
ways in which women had been separated from each other by men.
Sisterhood was emphasised as a way of establishing solidarity and
unity and as a means of challenging common bonds of discrimination and oppression. However, within feminism, black women
and white working class women found difficulty in espousing
common cause with perspectives which were seen to reflect white
women's middle class concerns. Differences, in relation to forms
of disadvantage, discrimination and oppression emerged, as did
factors associated with different social, cultural, racial and economic
circumstances.

Disability rights movements based on the social model of disability have also emphasised unity rather than diversity. As highlighted in Chapter 3, there are those such as Begum (1992), Morris
(1993a) and Crow (1996) who from within the social model of
disability want to explore differences related to gender, age, 'race',

ethnicity and impairment. There are others such as Oliver (1996) and Finkelstein (1993a) who are wary of the consequences of exploring these areas, because of the implications for the unity of the movement and the coherence of the social model. This stance has political advantages in terms of pressing for rights-based citizenship entitlements for disabled people, but a disadvantage could be seen to be an assumed homogeneity. As with feminism(s), assumed and projected similarities can lead to challenge and fragmentation.

Chapter 3 explores how problems and developments within disability rights movements can be seen to be mirroring problems and developments within feminist movements. However, at this stage the difficulties associated with projected homogeneity have considerable relevance and lead on to the question: who qualifies as a disabled person?

With regard to the social model of disability, all those who are discriminated against by others on the basis of perceived impairments would be seen to qualify as disabled people. However, this is far from straightforward, as is demonstrated by the case of ME (or myalgic encephalomyelitis). ME is a condition that impairs, but this is an impairment that may not be recognised by others. Disabling processes in this instance can be seen to be twofold in that initially an individual has to fight to be accepted as disabled; once accepted they then have to contend with the difficulties associated with living in a disabling society. There are also universalising gender stereotypes to consider. Some disabling perspectives, for example, can regard disability as being more psychologically acceptable for a woman than for a man, in that a woman can be seen to be more conditioned to accept dependency and passivity. To return to the example of ME, prevailing differential expectations placed on men and women could result in the condition being regarded as more socially and culturally acceptable in a woman than in a man.

Overall, with regard to the question 'who qualifies as a disabled person?' unitary categorisations on the basis of frequently changing qualifying criteria used by government agencies and assumed unities related to the experience of discrimination used by 'second wave' feminists and disability rights organisations, can be seen to result in the contradiction which can best be expressed as a standardised lack of clarity. Put simply, 'disability' is a contested concept and, accordingly, there can be no clear answer to the question posed.

Writing about disability issues: who should do it?

Writing about disability is a far from straightforward process and raises issues relating to knowledge production and political intent. The social model of disability, which will be discussed in greater detail in Chapter 2, has as its central proposition the view that we all have impairments, some more obvious than others, but that disability is an oppressive social construct (e.g. Oliver 1983, 1990, 1996; Barnes 1990, 1997; Barton and Oliver 1997; Barnes et al. 1999).[2] Emphasis is placed on overcoming disabling barriers in a move away from 'cure and care' scenarios which concentrate on individual impairments (Finkelstein 1993b). Many supporters of the social model of disability are critical of non-disabled writers publishing material relating to disability. There is the fear that disabled people will be exploited, that the material will have academic relevance only and that non-disabled writers cannot connect with the 'standpoint' of disabled people. These are valid and important concerns, but they also raise further questions; for example, is it the experience of disability that is important, or the mediation and theorisation of experience?

With regard to the question of whether it is the experience of disability that is important or the mediation and theorisation of experience, Barton (1996) and Moore et al. (1998), who discuss this topic in the context of research, suggest that it is a writer's orientation and commitment to disability issues that is crucial and that the experience of being disabled is important but not imperative. In this context, it is useful to pre-empt the discussion in Chapter 3 and to highlight the similarities between 'second wave' feminist movements and disability movements. Although the context is different, the privileging of experience can be seen to be a key feature of both. In relation to disability rights movements based on the social model of disability, experience of disability is often seen as the only means of establishing credibility. Within feminism(s), the use of essentialist experiential accounts was viewed as a way of countering universalising tendencies and of deconstructing the category 'woman'. However, it was subsequently questioned on the basis that it proved divisive and raised issues about who had the most right to speak as a feminist. Maynard (1994), for example, maintains that although women's experiences can be regarded as a starting point for the production of feminist knowledge, experience alone cannot help in understanding the processes and practices that have to be seen as constituent parts of feminist epistemologies or knowledge frameworks. She asserts:

> To repeat and describe what women might have to say, while important, can lead to individualisation and fragmentation, instead of analysis. Feminism(s) has an obligation to go beyond citing experience in order to make connections which may not be visible from the purely experiential level alone. This is an interpretative and synthesising process which connects experience to understanding.
>
> (Maynard 1994: 23–4)

With regard to experience, there are also criticisms that the social model of disability overlooks detail in favour of emphasising its overall agenda. Stalker (1998) maintains in relation to people with learning difficulties that:

> the social model of disability 'creates a vision' whereby it is possible to imagine a group of people with learning difficulties getting together themselves, identifying the need for a research project, designing it, employing interviewers and overseeing its execution, or even doing it themselves. In other words, the social model implies that all that is wanting before people with learning difficulties are able to take control of the research process is to overcome certain disabling barriers. This view rests on an analysis of disability as a function of material, social, economic and cultural barriers.
>
> (Stalker 1998: 15)

The issue of 'impairment' is explored in greater detail in Chapter 2, but it is important to emphasise here, the ways in which discussions about impairment serve as points of critique for the social model of disability.

To illustrate the point further it is also useful to change the emphasis slightly. I am a woman and although there are points of similarity at a structural level between barriers that I and other women face, our experiences will be different. I could claim that my experiences are more valid because I feel I have experienced greater oppression or I could contend that my experiences are more representative than those of others, but this, unsurprisingly, is likely to be regarded as a contentious and unsustainable claim. Accordingly, it would be difficult for me to claim that on the basis of my experiences I could speak for all women. On a slightly different note, as a feminist, I support many feminist political campaigns, but in terms of strategy, would I bar pro-feminist men from writing about feminism(s) and associated political campaigns? As with all illustrations, the issues have been very simply put, but the underlying arguments remain and require consideration.

It is therefore possible to argue that personal experiences are important, but that they are not enough when it comes to amassing a body of knowledge that has to be theoretical as well as personal. The formation and constitution of the social model of disability, for example, clearly highlights that generalising and theorising processes featured significantly, with experience being regarded as a necessary but specific and mediated component. There are also points of comparison with debates in relation to 'race' and gender. A key point made by writers in these fields is the need to theorise from experience, to avoid reductionism and to examine the interrelationship and interaction between the individual and society, taking full account of the operation of power and the creation of social divisions (e.g. Barrett 1987; Brah 1992; Gilroy 1992; Williams 1992; Fawcett 1996a).

To return to the point made by Barton (1996) and Moore et al. (1998) and the question about who should write about disability, perhaps rather than sole emphasis being placed on experiences of disability, issues of reflexivity and process should be considered. Accordingly, points of interrogation such as 'Why am I undertaking this project?', 'What is its purpose?' and 'How might my values and belief systems influence the project?' become key.

These are questions which need to be addressed in the context of this book. Firstly with regard to 'Why am I undertaking this project?' I have to point to my own experiences, which span personal, professional and academic arenas, of working in the area of disability and to my engagement over the years with feminism(s) in its many and varied forms. These experiences are context-specific and when reviewed from the perspective of the present, highlight ongoing concerns with the attainment of full citizenship rights for oppressed groupings coupled with a simultaneous emphasis on issues of difference and diversity. It also has to be stated that I have no desire to present another contesting model or theory, or to imply that I have insights into 'disability' which others lack. My aim is not to appropriate debates, but to contribute to a full and lively discussion.

In this context, my purpose in writing this book has been to examine the similarities between current disability rights movements based on the social model of disability and feminist movements. In particular I want to explore the tensions between the projection of a unitary front to serve political ends and the needs of movement members to celebrate diversity and difference. My intention is also, through the introduction in Chapter 5 of perspectives drawn from postmodern feminism(s), to look at ways in which issues of difference and diversity can be explored and responded to without resulting in fragmentation and schism.

With regard to the ways in which my values and belief systems might influence this project, I have been profoundly influenced by the social model of disability. Its importance in terms of facilitating constructive challenges to negative conceptualisations of disability and disabling images and the ways in which it has generated a reappraisal of services and organisations based on a particular view of disabled people, has to be both emphasised and applauded. As discussed above, there are problem areas related to the exploration of dimensions such as gender, 'race', age, class and impairment and these areas are appraised in Chapters 2 and 3. Nevertheless wide-ranging changes have occurred as a result of the social model of disability and its significance has to be fully acknowledged.

In relation to my ontological and epistemological position, or how I view the world and my knowledge base, I have to state at this stage that I have been strongly influenced by postmodern feminist perspectives. These are discussed in Chapter 5, but suffice it to say here that such perspectives reject views of knowledge as objective and value-free. Similarly the 'big stories' emanating from that eighteenth-century phenomena known as the Enlightenment, relating to an overriding believe in progress, reason and the possibility of accessing 'the truth', are eschewed. Instead, there is an emphasis on deconstruction, that is critically interrogating taken for granted knowledge frameworks and of accepting that all knowledge claims, even those emanating from oppressed groupings, are partial. The notion of subjects and subjectivity as coherent, integrated and unique also gives way to an emphasis on process, fluidity and change. Postmodern feminist perspectives are also generally critical of the relativity and pluralism of postmodern writers such as Lyotard (1984). Orientations drawn from postmodern feminism(s) variously present reformulations whereby postmodern social criticism can reject foundationalism (or the unquestioning acceptance of an established principle or premise) and the 'metanarratives' of the Enlightenment whilst retaining a form of contextual grounding, which facilitates the recognition of social differences and divisions and the weighting of criteria in relation to concepts of justice, equity and fairness (Fraser and Nicholson 1993; Fawcett 1998).

Concluding remarks

At this point it is also pertinent to outline the structure of the book as a whole. This chapter, as highlighted above, looks at who should write about disability and considers matters of gender. Chapter 2 critically appraises debates relating to 'individual' or 'medical' and 'social' models of disability and the relationship of these models to essentialist and constructionist debates. The place of individual impairment is also considered in this context. The impact of categorising processes in relation to disability, raised initially in Chapter 1, is also explored further in Chapter 2. Notions of risk and risk assessment are additionally reviewed as part of this discussion. Chapter 3 returns to a key theme introduced in Chapter 1, relating to the notion of experience and whether an individual can only write about what they have experienced. It explores the links between disability rights movements based on the social model of disability and feminist movements. In this chapter, feminist analyses are used both as a point of comparison and as a critical tool. Chapter 4 examines current community care policies and, by means of an appraisal of associated opportunities and constraints, assesses the impact of these upon women and upon disabled women and men. Issues relating to private and public arenas and concepts of citizenship, as constituting the interface between, are also explored. Chapter 5 looks at what is meant by postmodernism and explores conceptualisations of postmodern feminism(s). Some of the areas considered in Chapter 3 are re-appraised from postmodern feminist perspectives and aspects related to power/knowledge frameworks, notions of subjectivity, matters of difference and conceptualisations of able-bodiedness, disabled-bodiedness and the body, are particularly highlighted. Finally, Chapter 6 explores how orientations drawn from postmodern feminism(s) could be applied to the field of disability and how these orientations could contribute towards an inclusive, rather than an exclusive, approach.

The book overall, by drawing from postmodern feminism(s), emphasises that 'disability' has personal, social, historical, cultural and textual components. It highlights that although there are many ways of viewing disability, with none able to claim absolute validity, strategic groupings and alliances promulgating perspectives which challenge engendered categorisations, dogma, stereotypes and processes of subordination, can effectively achieve wide-ranging changes for disabled women and men.

Summary

- Writing about disability has been seen as highly contentious. Questions relating to discussions about whether only disabled people can write about disability and the place of gender in such discussions, have been considered.

- The various and varying feminist perspectives have been reviewed and the term 'feminism(s)' coined to refer to all the perspectives contained within 'feminism'.

- The ways in which 'disabled people' and 'women' are often seen to comprise undifferentiated, unitary groupings have been examined and matters of difference and diversity highlighted.

- The place of experience in discussions about disability has been explored and the utility of mediating and theorising from experience has been emphasised.

- The ways in which 'appropriation' or the taking over of issues, discussion and debates that involve disabled women and men, have been reviewed.

- A summary has been given of the overall structure of this book.

Notes

1 Postmodernism, postmodern feminism(s) and the deconstruction of gender is discussed in Chapter 5.

2 The social model of disability is discussed in detail in Chapter 2.

Further reading

Barnes, C. and Mercer, G. (eds) (1997) *Doing Disability Research*, Leeds: The Disability Press.

Barnes, C., Mercer, G. and Shakespeare, T. (1999) *Exploring Disability: A Sociological Introduction*, Cambridge: Polity Press.

Barrett, M. and Phillips, A. (1992) (eds) *Destabilising Theory: Contemporary Feminist Debates*, Cambridge: Polity Press.

Barton, L. (1996) (ed.) *Disability and Society: Emerging Issues and Insights,* London: Longman.

Barton, L. and Oliver, M. (1997) (eds) *Disability Studies: Past, Present and Future,* Leeds: The Disability Press.

Bock, L. and James, S. (eds) (1992) *Beyond Equality and Difference,* London: Routledge.

Brah, A. (1992) 'Difference, Diversity and Differentiation' in Donald, J. and Rattansi, A. (eds) *'Race', Culture and Difference,* London: Sage, Open University Press.

Moore, M., Beazley, S. and Maelzer, J. (1998) *Researching Disability,* Buckingham: Open University Press.

Chapter 2

'Disability': a contested topic

Chapter outline

This chapter focuses on the following:

- the ways in which disabled people have been positioned over time
- individual or medical models of disability
- the social model of disability
- categorising processes
- notions of risk and risk assessment
- self-categorising processes

Introduction

Busfield (1996), looking at gender and mental disorder in the context of the nineteenth century, writes:

> What we observe is a set of assumptions not just about biological difference, but about the biological weakness and vulnerability of the female, with a typical gender asymmetry: the supposedly general account of human biological functioning is assumed to apply to the male but not to the female who is held to require special considerations. In this way, the male is positioned as normal, the female as some deviation.
>
> (Busfield 1996: 146)

Shakespeare (1994), drawing from Simone de Beauvoir (1953), asserts in relation to disabled people:

If original sin, through the transgression of Eve, is concretized
in the flesh of woman, then the flesh of disabled people has
historically, and within Judeo-Christian theology especially,
represented divine punishment for ancestral transgression.

(Shakespeare 1994: 292)

The positionings of women and disabled women and men have
varied over recorded time relating to prevailing economic circumstances, hierarchical status, personal characteristics, the orientations
of particular societies, the cultural dictates of the time and the
direction of the religious teachings or belief systems. At times, binary stances have been adopted and these are particularly apparent
with regard to religion. Accordingly, disabled children have been
regarded as changelings and taken as evidence of the mother's
involvement in sorcery or witchcraft. They have also been seen
as a means of demonstrating Christian charity and compassion.
Similarly women have been viewed as symbols of purity and per-
fection, as in the Virgin Mary, or as wanton temptresses. However,
although there have been variations, it also appears that women and
disabled women and men have been regarded as being different
from dominant groupings of men. This difference has often carried
with it negative, rather than positive connotations.

Shakespeare (1994), as indicated above, applies the analysis of
how women have been regarded as 'other', closely associated with
nature, and viewed as being in need of guidance and control, to
disabled people. Accordingly normality is confirmed by being compared to abnormality or the 'other'.[1] Devalued groupings by default
confirm the valuation of other groupings. Shakespeare (1994) suggests that the identity of individuals is strengthened by the isolation
and rejection of anomaly or difference. A definition of normality
must rest on a definition of abnormality. Shakespeare, drawing
from Douglas (1966), asserts:

When boundaries are breached, and identities seem threatened,
behaviour is devoted to re-establishing the fixates, reinforcing
categories and power relations.

(Shakespeare 1994: 294)

Shakespeare further maintains:

This underlies the difference between having an impairment
(a common experience) and being disabled (a specific social
identity of a minority): or between various sexual practices, and
between specific gay and straight identities.

(Shakespeare 1994: 294–5)

Shakespeare refers to people with impairments as 'the ultimate non-conformists' and as 'perpetually threatening to the self image of the average, so called "normal" population' (Shakespeare 1994: 296).

Shakespeare (1994) extends his analysis to cultural representations and he highlights the ways in which women and disabled people are objectified in culture. He asserts that such objectification carries with it demeaning images akin to processes of colonisation and imperialism. He maintains that cultural 'objectifications' affect daily social interaction and, drawing from Hevey (1992), states that 'everyday interaction for disabled people involves an invasion, by "normal" people, of disabled people' (Shakespeare 1994: 288). Accordingly disabled people are continually objectified by the reaction of others; reactions which include staring, pity and hostility (Morris 1993a).

In this chapter, essentialist and constructionist definitions of disability, associated in turn with individual (or medical) and social models of disability, will be examined. Objectifying categorisation processes will be explored and consideration given to the utility of self-categorisation processes for disabled women and men. Finally, following on from an appraisal of categorising processes and the impact of these, notions of risk and risk assessment will be critically reviewed. As discussed in Chapter 1, 'disability' is a contested area and definitions of disability vary according to historical context, cultural and social location and the nature of the environment. The aim of this chapter is to explore the contested nature of disability, placing emphasis on current perspectives.

Individual or medical models of disability

Before examining the social model of disability in greater detail, it is useful to explore its binary opposite – the 'individual' or medical model of disability. Both models can be regarded as forming opposing parts of the same frame. Oliver, who can be seen as one of the primary instigators of the social model of disability, originally used the term 'individual model' (Oliver 1983: 15) to refer to the 'medicalisation' of disability (Oliver 1996: 31). However, as Oliver (1996) points out, the 'individual' model was rapidly followed by the formulation of a number of other models variously termed 'medical', 'psychological', 'charity' and 'administrative' models.[2] All of these models can be seen to have been influenced by notions of biological determinism and all focus on medically orientated 'cure and care' agendas. Over time these different models, in terms of both label and content, have become conflated and the term 'medical models' is now frequently used to refer to the 'medicalisation' of disability.

According to the social model of disability, any conceptualisation of disability that does not view 'disability' as an oppressive social construct and highlight socio-cultural understandings, can be regarded as coming under the umbrella of 'medical model' frameworks. Prior to the emergence of the social model, both theoretical and applied understandings of 'disability', which focused on classifying impairments and regarding impairment as an individual experience, were generally accepted as 'the' way to understand disability. The hegemonic or dominant position afforded to this perspective of disability can be analysed by way of the 'three-dimensional' operation of power described by Lukes (1974: 23). He asserts:

> Is it not the supreme and most invidious exercise of power to prevent people from having grievances by shaping their perceptions in such a way that they accept their role in the existing order of things, either because they can see or imagine no alternative, or because they see it as natural and unchangeable, or because they value it as divinely ordained and beneficial?
>
> (Lukes 1974: 24)

The overall acceptance of the medicalised framework can also be compared to Foucault's conception of the dominant discourse (Foucault 1981a). As will be discussed in greater detail in Chapter 5, Foucault uses the term 'discourse' to examine how power, language and institutional practices combine at historically specific points in time to determine modes of thought. The amount of power exercised by the various discourses relates to the ways in which meaning, knowledge and therefore 'truth' is appropriated, or to put it another way, the extent to which dominant discourses define conceptions of normality. Foucault argues that people can only understand or conceptualise from within discourses and that people are both the subjects and agents of competing discourses (Foucault 1979, 1981a,b; Foucault, in Gordon 1980).[3] For example, a woman might be subject to the competing discourses emanating from 'medical models' of disability, the social model and the various feminism(s), with all these discourses prescribing competing projects around feminism and disability. According to Foucault, there are also contradictions within discourses which carry the possibility of resistance and the formulation of alternative discourses. Here, arguably dominant modes of conceptualising disability have always carried seeds of alternative discourses, which could be seen to have resulted in the emergence of the social model of disability.

Both the perspectives of Lukes and Foucault have their critics and there will be a further examination of power/knowledge frameworks in Chapter 5 in relation to an exploration of postmodern feminism(s). However, a brief discussion of the dominant position and the institutional sanction afforded to the medicalisation of disability is useful at this point in that it establishes the basis for later discussions.

At this stage it is pertinent to look at the medicalisation of disability in more detail and to consider varying explanations and perspectives. To draw again from Foucault (1979), he saw the era from the seventeenth century onwards as being part of the creation of the 'disciplinary society'. Foucault (1979) argues that about this time there was a shift from sovereign power, which was episodic and brutal in terms of punishment being directly inflicted upon the body of the caught 'criminal', to disciplinary power, which is more pervasive in that it is ever present, regulatory and routinised. Sovereign power was related to notions of personal service and reward for the upper classes, who in turn managed the populace in their locality by means of a system of dues, obligations and personal punishments. People by and large knew their place and, apart from military endeavours, tended to remain in their locality. The impetus for the shift from sovereign power to disciplinary power has been seen by Bauman (1992) and Clegg (1992) to have been set in motion by a gradual shift from feudal rights to property rights, population pressure and by the increasing mobility of the population.

Disciplinary power, according to Foucault, resulted in the formation of new forms of surveillance and containment. The operation of disciplinary institutions and disciplinary power in this context can be seen to have drawn from existing institutions such as the monasteries. Bentham's Panopticon, a building which he devised in the nineteenth century, comprising a central all-seeing tower surrounded by a circular system of constantly lit cells, typified for Foucault the operation of disciplinary power. Here inmates would be under constant surveillance and would eventually, through an appreciation that there was no getting away from the all-seeing but unseen eye, surveill themselves. The Panopticon can be seen to represent a trend, a means of control transferred to the population at large and reinforced by institutions such as the Church, the State and its legislature, schools, factory systems and the family. As Clegg

points out, disciplinary power represented 'disciplined subordination' (Clegg 1992: 175). Those who would or could not discipline
themselves, or who were different, physically or mentally, were
subject to dividing practices, which created the divisions healthy/
ill, sane/mad, legal/delinquent and, it is possible to add, able-
bodied/disable-bodied. Foucault states:

> dividing practices separate and objectify people from social groups
> for exhibiting difference. The actions of dividing practices are made
> acceptable by claims of science and the institutional backing given
> to the operation of scientific discourses. This in turn can be seen to
> lead to scientific classification and categorisation.
> (Foucault, cited in Gordon 1980: 65)

Institutions such as the workhouse and the large bureaucratised
asylums contained and controlled those deemed incapable of
operating in accordance with accepted tenets and surveilling and
disciplining themselves. The asylums became increasingly medicalised and also incorporated, in line with the emphasis placed on
scientific endeavour and progress, a curative function. As Merquior
(1985) points out, madness in particular became a disease. As far
as Foucault (1979) was concerned, this led to the control of 'un-
reason' and to moral and mental as well as physical imprisonment.
For individuals regarded as 'different', medical practices became
the ultimate form of surveillance.

Other writers present differing explanations for the increasing
dominance of medical perspectives in relation to disability. Scull
(1979), for example, from a Marxist perspective, relates the rise
of medicalisation to the expansionist and financially influenced
motivations of medical professionals who seized the opportunity
presented to them by industrialisation, urbanisation and the prevailing scientific ideology of the nineteenth century. Barnes (1997a)
in turn claims that the nineteenth century, for a whole variety of
reasons, including industrialisation, the break-up of the extended
family, population increases, mobility, belief in scientific endeavour,
eugenics and so on, can be seen as synonymous with the emergence
of 'disability' in its twentieth-century, individually and medically
orientated form.

This individually and medically orientated form, where emphasis
is placed on individual impairments and classification systems,
according to the social model of disability, leaves disabled people
with a limited number of positions to occupy. They can either strive
to overcome their disability and paradoxically aspire to a 'normality'
which they will never attain, or accept their status as an object of

pity and of fear; an object that can be related to able-bodiedness in terms of: 'I'm so relieved that isn't me, but I fear ending up like that'. With regard to fear, Longmore (1987) draws attention to how able-bodied individuals 'often stigmatise and shun and sometimes seek to destroy' that which is feared (Longmore 1987: 66) and this is an area which, although often ignored, can be seen to have featured significantly in the treatment of disabled people both culturally and historically. In terms of responses, again these are seen to be limited with various permutations of 'care and control' applying (Oliver 1983, 1990, 1993, 1996; Barnes 1990, 1997b;[4] Swain *et al.* 1993; Barton 1996).

At this point it is also useful to consider the 'socio-medical model' of disability (Bury 1996). This is a model which focuses on the social dimensions of medicalised conceptions of disability, and which in terms of content, can be seen to have additional areas to highlight. Barnes (1997a) maintains that this model of disability has its roots in the 1940s work of Talcott Parsons and the functionalist school of sociology, which saw sickness and, by implication, impairment as deviations from normality. Bury (1996) asserts that this emphasis continued into the 1960s and 1970s, resulting in collaborative work between sociology and medicine which focused on estimating medical need and the development of preventative strategies. Examples here include the work of Harris *et al.* (1971) whose studies were also associated with the formulation of the Chronically Sick and Disabled Persons Act (1970). This work resulted in calls for the clarification of the terminology used, and the International Classification of Impairments, Disabilities and Handicaps was published by the World Health Organisation in 1980 (Wood 1980). In this document, 'impairment' was defined as abnormality, 'disability' as restricted abilities in relation to self-care and everyday tasks, and 'handicap' was defined as social disadvantage that could be associated with either impairment or disability. Despite the association of 'handicap' with disadvantage, the WHO definition can be seen to remain firmly rooted in medical classification systems (Oliver 1990).

The social model of disability

Individual or 'medical' models of disability are associated with individual pathologies, where emphasis is placed on cure or on the individual psychologically, physically and socially adjusting to their impairment. The social model of disability, in contrast, presents a structuralist, materially orientated analysis. Barnes (1997a) talks of the social model of disability as the socio–political approach which he sees as being influenced by two distinct but linked traditions. The first is seen to rely heavily on American functionalism and deviancy theory and points to the 'social construction' of the problem of disability as being an outcome of the evolution of contemporary society. The second, Barnes (1997a) sees as drawing from materialism and Marxism and regards disability and dependence as the 'social creation' of industrial capitalism (Barnes 1997a: 5).

The emergence of the social model of disability in the United Kingdom in particular, can be seen to be linked to the formation in the early 1970s of the Disablement Income Group, which later became the Disability Alliance and the Union of Physically Impaired Against Segregation (UPIAS). The history of these movements and the tensions between them are well documented by Finkelstein (1993b) and Oliver (1990, 1996) amongst others, and it is not pertinent to the current discussion to explore these in greater detail at this stage. However, in 1976 the key *Fundamental Principles of Disability* document was published by UPIAS and this marked a crucial juncture in relation to disability research, political activity and theoretical debate. This document rejected the representation of disabled people by 'experts' and re-defined disability. Oliver's 1996 edited version of the 1976 document states:

> In our view, it is society which disables physically impaired people.
> Disability is something imposed on top of our impairments by
> the way we are unnecessarily isolated and excluded from full
> participation in society. Disabled people are therefore an oppressed
> group in society. To understand this it is necessary to grasp the
> distinction between the physical impairment and the social situation,
> called 'disability', of people with such impairment. Thus we define
> impairment as lacking part of or all of a limb, or having a defective
> limb, organ or mechanism of the body; and disability as the
> disadvantage or restriction of activity caused by a contemporary
> social organisation which takes no or little account of people
> who have physical impairments and thus excludes them from
> participation in the mainstream of social activities. Physical disability
> is therefore a particular form of social oppression.
>
> (Oliver 1996: 22)

The Disabled People's International (DPI) use 'disability' and 'handicap' instead of 'impairment' and 'disability' but the associations are the same.

The social model of disability, sometimes called the social barriers model of disability, embraces the definition of disability outlined above. It emphasises the segregationist, disablist (in that scientific objectivity is claimed which gives qualified professionals control over disabled people) and dependency creating implications of 'medical models' for disabled people. Research into disability based on WHO definitions, OPCS surveys[5] and medical activity are found to be inadequate and oppressive. Medical models are critiqued for focusing on the specific condition, with medically orientated classification and administrative systems being regarded as encouraging slippage into the person becoming the condition: for example, an individual becomes 'a paraplegic' who then becomes part of a grouping called 'paraplegics' with homogeneous characteristics assumed. Oliver asserts that the power and dominance of the medical profession has 'spawned a whole range of pseudo professions in its own image . . . each one geared to the same aim – the restoration of normality' (Oliver 1996: 37).

The social model focuses on attitudinal and physical constraints. Disability is not regarded as the problem of the individual, but as a social and environmental issue. An individual is therefore not disabled by their specific condition, but by external restraints which prevent them from living their life in the way that they would want. Oliver (1990) maintains that the social model is based upon social constructionist and social creationist perspectives. He regards both as contributing to the barriers faced by disabled people, but regards the social constructionist view as locating the problem 'within the minds of able-bodied people, whether individually (prejudice) or collectively, through the manifestation of hostile social attitudes and the enactment of social policies based upon a tragic view of disability' (Oliver 1990: 82). The social creationist view places the problem within the institutionalised practices of society (Oliver 1990: 83). Oliver uses this distinction to argue for legislative changes and for the orientation to be about changes in behaviour rather than attitudes. He argues that the discredited 'awareness' training exercises of the early 1980s proved unsuccessful and unpopular because they just concentrated on negative individual and social attitudes rather than upon the operating practices of powerful organisations and institutions. The point is well made, but others would perhaps question the social constructionist and social creationist distinction (e.g. Payne 1991; Harvey 1992).

Shakespeare (1996) maintains that the social model of disability is only one way of identifying disability as a social process and that there are three others. Although supportive of the overall agenda of the social model, he is critical of its broad-brush approach whereby disabled people can be seen as one group amongst many who experience disabling barriers. With regard to other related models, the minority group approach Shakespeare maintains often co-exists with the social model and highlights issues of oppression, power and identity politics. Shakespeare argues that according to his definition, the first model, the social model, can be regarded as a social constructionist model, whereas the second model, the minority group approach, particularly with its focus on identity politics, carries with it the potential to reinforce the categorisation of disabled people as a separate group. The third model, the Weberian or Foucauldian approach, according to Shakespeare, sees disability as a category of social policy which serves to move attention away from the individual with an impairment to the policy processes whereby the individual is constructed as 'officially' disabled. Within this approach, 'disability' is seen as the outcome of social research definitions. Accordingly, the ways in which OPCS categories, for example, are arbitrarily constructed, yet the resultant totals of disabled people recorded as official fact, are emphasised. Finally and fourthly, disability as a cultural category highlights how processes of denial and projection are involved in the cultural constitution of disability. Shakespeare (1994) calls for the social model to be further developed to take into account not just material discrimination, but also prejudice reflected in cultural representation, language and socialisations, which resonate at the interpersonal level.

Shakespeare's elaboration of the varying ways in which disability can be seen as a social process highlights an important issue and one which warrants further attention at this point. This relates to the ways in which social constructionism can be defined. Social constructionism refers to a broad area and Burr (1995) identifies four key assumptions which can be regarded as common to all social constructionist writings. These are: the critical interrogation of taken-for-granted knowledge; that ways of understanding are seen as embedded in specific historical, cultural and social time periods and relate to the particular circumstances of the period; that knowledge is a result of social processes; and that interactions and understandings or knowledge frames and social action are linked. An example, and one highlighted in the discussions in this chapter, is that different understandings of disability produce different responses.

However, although there are similarities there are also differences between, for example, the social constructionist approach adopted by Berger and Luckmann (1966) and poststructural or postmodern[6] understandings which highlight discursive positionings and how subjects are positioned in discourse. The former focuses on how an externalised idea or practice, such as the view that women should not work but stay at home with their children, becomes an object of consciousness. Accordingly, such an idea or practice takes on a momentum of its own and becomes accepted to the extent that it is then internalised into the consciousness of the next generation as an existing and irrefutable given. Discursive positionings, in contrast, tend to draw from French philosophical traditions, particularly the work of Foucault, and concentrate on how different groups in society are positioned differently with regard to particular discourses. For example, women are positioned differently to men within a discourse of gender. Within a gendered discourse, the position of disabled women is also different to that of able-bodied women.

In the United Kingdom, the social model of disability is closely linked to disability rights campaigns. These campaigns focus on enforceable equal rights legislation, for the social model of disability to form the basis for professional and institutional interaction with disabled people, for funding to organisations *of* rather than organisations *for* disabled people and full citizenship. The Americans with Disabilities Act 1990 has been cited as a progressive piece of legislation and one to which the United Kingdom should aspire. The Disability Discrimination Act 1995, which was introduced in a piecemeal fashion in Britain in 1996 and replaced defeated private member's bills on anti-discriminatory legislation for disabled people put forward by Roger Berry in 1994 and Harry Barnes in 1995, has been generally regarded as inadequate. It is seen as perpetuating 'medical model' understandings of disability and as requiring extensive revision. The Act does makes it illegal for the first time in the United Kingdom, to discriminate against disabled people with regard to employment, the provision of goods and services and the selling or letting of land or property (see Box 2.1). However, there are many opt-out clauses and, as stated above, definitions of disability remain firmly rooted in 'medical model(s)' classification systems which focus on the extent and duration of the disabilities experienced.

Oliver (1993, 1996) uses the work of T. H. Marshall (1952) to link citizenship with the achievement of political, social and civil

Box 2.1   Disability Discrimination Act 1995

The Disability Discrimination Act 1995 is set out in eight parts and is supplemented by eight schedules. The key provisions are as follows:

- The definitions that set out which people are covered by the Act. A disabled person is defined as a person 'who has a disability'. Disability is defined as a 'physical or mental impairment which has a substantial and long term adverse effect on a person's ability to carry out normal day to day activities'.
- The right for 'disabled people' not to be discriminated against in employment, unless there is a good reason. Employers employing under 20 people are exempt.
- The right for 'disabled people' not to be discriminated against in the supply of goods, facilities and services. However, this can be overturned if it can be argued that the health or safety of the disabled person or others would be in danger, or the customer is incapable of understanding the contract, or providing the service would deny service to other customers.
- The right for 'disabled people' not to be discriminated against in relation to selling or letting land or property.
- The provision of information for 'disabled people' by schools and further and higher educational establishments and local authorities.
- The setting of minimum standards for all new public transport vehicles.
- The establishment of a consultative National Disability Council and the Northern Ireland Disability Council.

rights. The disparity between full citizenship rights and the position of disabled people throughout society is then highlighted. Oliver argues and cites the Speaker's Commission on Citizenship (Department of Health 1990: xix) to support his position that there should be adequate minimum provision maintained by central government to ensure that all citizens can live in accordance with prevailing social standards. The provision of enforced anti-discrimination legislation would then ensure that disabled people could fully participate in society. Oliver maintains that disabled people need to be fully integrated into society. This view of citizenship is intended to be political and to serve as a focal point for change and as such lacks the analytical edge of writers such as Lister (1993, 1997), whose perspective is discussed in Chapter 4. Issues of gender are also not taken into account. However, this formulation of citizenship can be seen to support the social model and provide a useful rally-ing point for disability rights activists.

The social model of disability has also focused on language and terminology. The utility of the term 'disabled people' is highlighted, as this emphasises how people with impairments are disabled by society. Projected pejorative terms such as 'cripple', 'spastic', etc., are also being revalued and utilised in challenging ways by disabled people (Zola 1993). The revaluing of terms used previously as labels of abuse has been seen by many as a positive step, although Shake-speare (1996) points to the tensions associated with utilising a cat-egory created by others and to the dangers of a reconfirmation of difference sliding into essentialism and increased marginalisation. Accordingly, some writers have chosen to develop new terms. Wendell (1996), for example, is engaged on a project which focuses on emphasising difference rather than lack and she advocates a move away from a focus on 'corporeal inferiority' towards a positive reframing of disability as 'embodied difference'. In a similar fash-ion, deafness is also increasingly being re-termed 'linguistic differ-ence'. However, Finkelstein (1993a) in particular is critical of the latter move, believing it could result in a return to hierarchical categories of disability.

As previously mentioned, social constructionism applies to a very broad area and sometimes the distinctions highlighted above are emphasised, while at other times they are not. Within this very broad context, it is now useful to consider categorising processes and how these can be seen to apply to disabled people.

Categorising processes

As can be seen from the introduction to this chapter and from the examination of individual or 'medical models' and the social model of disability, perspectives and definitions of disability can be seen to be inextricably linked to categorising processes. Accepted social constructions, or taken-for-granted criteria, can be viewed as cat-egories which reflect dominant social and cultural groupings. These aspects can lead to categorising processes which project uniformity and define individuals or groups on the basis of simplistic, stereo-typical criteria usually for the purposes of administrative conveni-ence. Categorisation, as a process, can be applied to non-disabled as well as to disabled people. There is, nevertheless, a tendency for this process to be applied disproportionately to those who are seen to differ from what is expected. In Britain in particular, prefixes such as 'the' are used, leading to the commonplace usage of the term, 'the disabled'. This denies difference and diversity within groupings, whilst at the same time projecting negative assumptions. Categories, once constructed, can be uncritically accepted and can lead to those so categorised accepting associated negative valuations. Categorisation processes in relation to disabled people can have the effect of collapsing differences within and between women and men, so that others are required 'to speak for', 'to work on behalf of' and 'to look after' or 'to care for' those so categorised and to operate on the assumption that a physical impairment or impairments equals social, political and economic dysfunction and disqualification. It has also to be borne in mind that categorisation processes can be double-edged in that, as pointed out in Chapter 1, individuals not included within certain categorised groupings may have to fight to be included, for despite the frequent negative connotations, currently this can be the only way to obtain access to services.

As mentioned in the introduction to this chapter, there can also be similarities between social or projected categorising processes and the notion of 'the other' as used in feminist theory. As Wendell (1996) maintains, people are made 'other' by being regarded as a symbol of something which is feared or rejected. Disabled people are often seen by able-bodied people as 'other'; a group to be pitied, viewed with disgust, feared, because disabled people embody concerns held by able-bodied people about abnormal bodies, and above all regarded as a group which able-bodied people would not choose to be identified with. It also has to be borne in mind that people with disabilities can and do make each other become 'the other'. Said (1978), in a similar way to Shakespeare (1994), highlights the role played by differentiation in identity formation. This emphasises the ways in which individuals would view themselves in terms of their difference from someone else or another group. A study undertaken by the author (Fawcett 1999b), for example, showed how wheelchair users reacted angrily when seen by others as having a mental as well as a physical impairment.

Self-categorising processes

As a point of contrast, Jenness (1992) highlights the importance of self-categorising processes. She maintains that we all interpret our world in terms of social categories and that we choose to fit ourselves into the various categories recognised by the community. However, such categories are reconstructed by individuals to take account of idiosyncratic factors and as such are divested of stereotypical attributes. Jenness (1992) maintains that there is an ongoing interrelationship between identity creation and self-categorisation processes.

Projected categorisation processes, which often carry associated social stigma, can be seen to reduce the options and the personal choices of disabled people, rendering the creative self-categorisation process outlined by Jenness (1992), fraught and difficult. However, the social model of disability has been seen by many disabled people as a basis for rejecting projected negative categorisations. According to Venkatesh (1993), it has enabled disabled people to engage in the process of self-discovery.

Edwards (1994) draws attention to the continuity across time and space of the oppression of disabled people and a key issue to address at this point relates to why 'disability' carries with it such negative connotations. Biological/medical classification systems which use a definition of normality as a starting point and identify deviation on the basis of a categorical index of impairments, as outlined, have been seen as having a major part to play in this process (e.g. Oliver 1990; Barnes 1990, 1997b; Shakespeare 1996, amongst many others). Prevailing ideologies, which include the religious, the individualistic and the materialistic, can also be seen to have played a part. Shakespeare (1996), however, changes the parameters of such a discussion and, drawing from OPCS surveys and highlighting that although there are differences of degree, everybody has impairments of one sort or another, asks why 'able-bodied' people ignore their physical limitations. He asserts:

> Perhaps the maintenance of a non disabled identity in the context of physical limitation is a more useful problem with which to be concerned: rather than interrogating the other, let us rather deconstruct the normality-which-is-to-be-assumed.
>
> (Shakespeare 1996: 96)

The creation of categories produces individuals to fill these categories (Hacking 1986) and, as highlighted above, categorisation processes can be seen to be related to the process of identity creation. As discussed, current debates in the arena of disability are dominated by 'medical models' versus the social model of disability polarisations. 'Medical models' are regarded by proponents of the social model of disability as promoting negative concepts of self-identity, dominated by the linkage of impairment and deficiency and associated with notions of loss, limitations and adjustment.

The social model of disability highlights negative social relations, not impairment, and emphasises different ways of viewing the self. However, although the social model of disability moves the focus away from individual impairments viewed as limitations, there can still be seen to be an emphasis on the limitations placed on an individual by the ways in which society and non-disabled individuals, disable. Accordingly, a disabled individual can be seen to be oppressed either by their impairment or by social barriers and although the latter can be associated with the development of challenging responses, it can also be linked with the confirmation of victim status. Overall, the categorisations available which can be used positively are far less extensive than those available to an able-bodied individual.

Shakespeare (1996), exploring issues concerning disabled people and identity formation, highlights the concept of identity as narrative as a useful way of avoiding linking identity straightforwardly with either medical or social constructs. Shakespeare stresses his commitment to understanding 'disability' as a social construction and to emphasis placed by the social model of disability on material, environmental and policy factors. However, he rejects a reductionist perspective which views the category 'disability' straightforwardly as a social relation and highlights the importance of complexity and difference and of linking political, cultural and personal aspects of disability.

Shakespeare (1996) and also Thomas (1999) point to the utility of placing emphasis on the stories we tell about ourselves and our lives, and on the importance of constructing accounts which encompass plot, causality and conflict. Shakespeare goes on to say that: 'This offers the potential for a nuanced model of identity which resists the temptation straightforwardly to read off identity for context, or indeed embodiment' (Shakespeare 1996: 99).

Shakespeare does not utilise orientations drawn from post-modern feminism(s) and there are differences between his perspective and those explored in Chapter 5. However, his project, which is to expand the horizons of the social model without moving away from the key tenets of the disability rights campaign, is one that contributes to debates and requires acknowledgement.

Notions of risk and risk assessment

In a discussion of disability, particularly one that reviews categorising and self-categorising processes, it is important to look at notions
of risk and risk assessment. In everyday speech, the term 'risk' is
often used in a non-specific way, and it can be unclear as to whether
it is risk to an individual who is considered vulnerable that is at issue
or the risk posed to the public by particular individuals. Currently,
with regard to these two areas, the former is often considered in
relation to individuals seen to have learning disabilities and the
latter to individuals with mental health problems. However, in the
nineteenth century and the first part of the twentieth century,
the asylum movement focused on protecting the public from all
individuals considered 'deficient' in some way. By means of the
exercise of control and care, emphasis was placed on protecting
the individual from risks perceived as dangers which they were considered unable to cope with.

With regard to definitions of risk, there is a focus on decisions
or courses of action having unintended consequences and as
Manthorpe *et al.* (1997) point out, risk is still often associated with
danger. This can overlook positive aspects of risk taking.

Heyman (1998) asserts that notions of risk in relation to health
and social care services are often seen as being externally quantifiable phenomena amenable to forms of cost–benefit analysis. He
cites the Royal Society (1992) as an influential force in promulgating this view which he associates with the application of a utilitarian
calculus. He states:

> The implicit or explicit calculation of expected value through cost–
> benefit analysis lies at the heart of a utilitarian rationality which
> enables general principles to be applied to concrete decision-making
> in science based cultures . . . Utilitarian reasoning attempts to
> combine scientific knowledge, expressed as probabilities, with value
> judgements in order to provide a rational basis for decision making.
>
> (Heyman 1998: 7–8)

His exposition of the process can be represented in the following
way. Alternative courses of action (or inaction) can be evaluated by
the identification of a set of practical choices. In relation to each
choice:

- the possible consequences are reviewed;
- a value which can be positive or negative is assigned to
  each consequence;

- the probability of each consequence occurring is estimated;
- the value of this choice is determined by looking at the values of the consequences in relation to their probabilities (based on Heyman 1998).

However, a key question to be asked is whether it is possible to assess risk in such a rational, objective and scientifically appropriate manner. Heyman and Henriksen (1998a) point out there are issues concerned with prediction, choice and value to take account of in relation to the assessment of risk and it is useful to consider these areas in more detail.

In order to subject risk to a cost–benefit analysis, it is important to be able to predict, on the basis of probability, that particular courses of action are associated with problematic or hazardous consequences. An examination of this area shows that such predictions are not as straightforward as might first appear and that historical context and historically located assumptions come into play. An example here relates to how in the nineteenth century female promiscuity among women from respectable families was viewed as a form of mental deficiency warranting incarceration in an institution. The consequences of not taking this course of action were regarded as morally and socially unacceptable both specifically with regard to the woman concerned, and generally, in relation to the family's perceived sense of duty. It was also believed in Britain in the 1950s that children of mixed race parentage were intellectually inferior to those who did not have mixed blood (Alibhai 1999). The risk of producing a 'mixed race' offspring was therefore viewed as a danger to be avoided.

With regard to matters of choice, it has to be appreciated that individuals may recognise something as hazardous, but not be able to, or choose to, or be too socially powerless to avoid it. Similarly, as Heyman and Henriksen (1998a) point out, actions can be seen to generate an infinite number of consequences. How these consequences are viewed can be associated with what is known, or what is investigated and valued. A woman might know, for example, that it is bad for her health to either under-eat or over-eat. However, conformity to a projected ideal of the perfect figure, or the need to obtain psychological sustenance by overindulging in certain desired food, may out-weigh a rational consideration of risk factors as a straightforward cost–benefit analysis implies. Similarly, cultural or social dictates related to smoking, drug-taking, body-piercing, etc., may take precedence over a clear-cut analysis of risks and benefits. With regard to probability, again Heyman and Henriksen (1998b) maintain:

> Users of the probability heuristic have to commit the ecological fallacy, attributing properties of groups defined for predictive purposes to individuals within those groups. The groupings which probabilistic prediction based on induction from observed frequencies has to draw on cannot, themselves, be defined unambiguously.
>
> (Heyman and Henriksen 1998b: 104)

In other words, it is far too simplistic to generalise from populations to individuals and to make what appear to be objective assertions on the grounds of inferred probability.

Overall then, the ways in which risks are viewed, the weighting attached to certain consequences, prevailing cultural and social values, the importance of specific contexts and contextual considerations and the ways in which these factors can overturn straightforward rational judgements, make risk assessment a more complicated process than might at first have been assumed. These areas are returned to in Chapter 6 when the contribution which orientations drawn from postmodern feminism(s) can make to the field of disability are appraised. However, at this point it is important to look at notions of risk and risk assessment in line with projected and self-categorising processes.

In this book, emphasis is placed on disability as a social construct, with some impairments being regarded as more exclusionary than others. For example, as highlighted by Manthorpe *et al.* (1997) in relation to learning disability, the Law Commission (1995) maintained that individuals whose mental capacity is severely impaired are not able to understand, retain or accept information, nor to reasonably foresee the results of their actions. Accordingly, the actions of all individuals with learning disabilities are seen to be qualitatively and quantitatively different from those who are not seen to have learning difficulties and who deliberately take risks with hazards attached. The generalisation contained in the Law Commission's pronouncement, when applied to diverse groupings of people, appears both discriminatory and oppressive. It is also far reaching, in that it forces professions to promote 'safety' both for the individual and the organisation, rather than to promote individual autonomy and choice. Assessments of risk can all too easily rely on simplistic definitions of words such as 'safety', the assumption of the mantle of rational control over another, and stereotypical generalisations.

Concluding remarks

This chapter has looked at the ways in which different definitions and conceptualisations of disability have resulted in disability becoming a contested area. However, the very nature of contestation and struggle can be seen to generate a dynamism that facilitates debate, action and change. The social model of disability has informed disability rights movements which have an emancipatory and liberatory agenda for disabled people. There are clear points of overlap here with 'second wave' feminist movements, and in Chapter 3 feminism will be used both as a point of comparison and as a critical tool to constructively interrogate both the social model of disability and emancipatory movements.

Summary

- The social model of disability has been considered in relation to its binary opposite, the individual or medical models of disability.

- Key features of individual or medical models include a focus on individual impairments and classification systems. An impairment is seen to be the problem of the individual.

- Key features of the social model include a focus on disabling attitudes, behaviours, environments and barriers generally. Oliver (1996) has invoked the concept of citizenship and has used it as a yardstick to draw attention to the lack of rights experienced by disabled people. The Disability Discrimination Act 1995 is not seen as going far enough in terms of barrier removal. The underlying philosophy of the Act is also seen to relate to an individual or medical models of disability rather than to the social model.

- The effect of the social model of disability on language use and the consequences of disabling social practices have been outlined. The varying models that can be seen to be associated with the social model, as detailed by Shakespeare (1996), have been discussed.

- Aspects of social constructionism have been briefly reviewed as a precursor to an exploration of categorising and self-categorising processes in relation to disability. It has been argued that with regard to both, disabled people are both positioned in a limited number of ways and have a limited number of positionings available to them.

• Notions of risk and risk assessment have been appraised and the ways in which risk can be defined and the utility of assessment procedures have been explored. It has been argued that often objectivity is erroneously assumed and that with regard to disabled women and men, risk is often associated with negative factors, rather than with positive opportunities. The way in which discourses of 'care and control' have been used to deny autonomy and choice have also been examined.

Notes

1 Simone de Beauvoir (1953: xvi) said that man is considered essential, woman inessential; man is 'the Subject', woman 'the Other'.

2 It is accepted that there are other models. The list given here is not meant to be definitive but to provide examples of models, which for the purposes of this book are being grouped under the heading 'medical models'.

3 By the use of 'subjects' and 'agents', Foucault generally (although he is not consistent) refers to how subjects are subjectified by discourses and also act as discursive agents in terms of perpetuating discursive practices.

4 This critique of 'medical models' draws from proponents of the social model of disability. The position adopted in this book is that it is not possible to appraise 'medical models' without drawing from critiques emanating from the social model of disability.

5 Classification systems such as the OPCS survey (1971) focused on functional assessments of disability which utilised a threefold distinction:

   (i)   impairment: lacking all or part of a limb or having a defective limb, organ or mechanism of the body;
   (ii) disablement: the loss or reduction of functional ability;
   (iii) handicap: the disadvantage or restriction of activity caused by the disability.

Responses to questions related to the capacity of individuals to care for themselves were grouped and disabled people divided into four categories:

(i)   very severely handicapped
(ii) severely handicapped
(iii) appreciably handicapped
(iv) impaired
(cited in Oliver 1983).

6 See Chapter 5 for a fuller discussion of poststructural and postmodern understandings.

Further reading

Barnes, C. and Mercer, G. (eds) (1996) *Exploring the Divide: Illness and Disability*, Leeds: The Disability Press.

Barnes, C., Mercer, G. and Shakespeare, T. (1999) *Exploring Disability: A Sociological Introduction*, Cambridge: Polity Press.

Barton, L. and Oliver, M. (eds) (1997) *Disability Studies: Past, Present and Future*, Leeds: The Disability Press.

Corker, M. and French, S. (eds) (1999) *Disability Discourses*, Buckingham: Open University Press.

Heyman, B. (ed.) (1998) *Risk, Health and Health Care*, London: Arnold.

Morris, J. (1993) *Pride Against Prejudice*, London: Women's Press.

Oliver, M. (1996) *Understanding Disability: From Theory to Practice*, Basingstoke: Macmillan.

Oliver, M. and Barnes, C. (1998) *Disabled People and Social Policy: From Exclusion to Inclusion*, London: Longman.

Swain, J., Finkelstein, V., French, S. and Oliver, M. (eds) (1993) *Disabling Barriers – Enabling Environments*, London: Open University Press/Sage.

Chapter 3

Feminism(s) and 'disability'

Chapter outline

In this chapter feminism(s) is used both as a point of comparison and as a tool to constructively critique the social model of disability. Key areas explored include the following:

- deconstructive analyses
- binary distinctions
- issues of unity
- the question of difference
- the place of experience
- disability and impairment
- disability and the body
- disability and oppression
- disability and standpoint positionings

Introduction

It is possible to assert that within the United Kingdom, the social model of disability and disability rights campaigns based on the social model of disability have only relatively recently begun to grapple with issues of difference and diversity between and amongst various groupings in relation to gender and also impairment, 'race', class, age, sexuality and varying dimensions of social division. Different writers within the field have adopted various positions. There are those within the disability movement, such as Oliver, who subsume issues of difference and diversity under the heading of 'multiple oppression' (Oliver 1996: 39). Oliver acknowledges the importance of this area, but is wary that greater exploration, particularly of impairment, may lead to fragmentation and disunity. There are others who support disability rights movements based on the social model of disability, but who critique the model for not considering gender, the effects of impairment and other differences. It is possible to assert that the most interesting critiques of the social model of disability have come from this grouping. French (1993) and Finkelstein (1993a), for example, have pointed out that within a broadly accepted political programme based on the social model of disability, certain areas such as disability benefits and the situation of older disabled people, particularly women and individuals with learning and communication impairments, continue to be contested. Begum (1992), Morris (1993a) and Abu-Habib (1997) have emphasised the need for a greater exploration of issues related to gender and 'race'. Morris (1993a), French (1993) and Crow (1996) have also specifically critiqued the social model of disability for appearing to ignore the implications of individual impairments. Shakespeare (1994), as highlighted in Chapter 2, argues for the social model to be reconceptualised to take into account not just material discrimination but prejudice which is implicit in cultural representation, language and socialisation. It is these critiques that will be built upon in this section.

Parallels have been drawn between feminism(s) and disability, in terms of theoretical positioning and with regard to the political and social message both have sought to convey. Comparisons have been made between rights based organisations of disabled people and black and feminist civil rights movements, and Shakespeare (1994) highlights the contribution made by feminist inspired writers towards the cultural representation of impairment.[1] A number of writers have also drawn attention to the utility of feminist perspectives, or have focused on gender distinctions in relation to disability.[2] However, arguably, none of the writers referred to above have sought to use feminism(s) both as a point of comparison and as a tool to constructively critique the social model of disability. This project will be the focus of this chapter with the key areas explored being those listed in the outline above. It also has to be pointed out that there will inevitably be some overlap with regard to the discussion of these key areas.

Deconstructive analyses

It is noteworthy that both the social model of disability and the varying feminisms deconstruct or critically interrogate taken-for-granted assumptions. With regard to feminism(s), this has led to white Western male notions of knowledge and language frameworks being recognised as value-laden. In relation to the social model of disability, this has resulted in the questioning of able-bodied knowledge claims and an exploration of the perspectives of disabled people. Abberley (1997), drawing from McKee (1982) and Hill Collins (1991), highlights the importance for disability movements of feminist deconstructive appraisals in relation to traditional policy solutions for dealing with inequality, poverty and employment.

Wendell (1996: 45) asserts that 'Much, but perhaps not all, of what can be socially constructed can be socially (and not just intellectually) deconstructed, given the means and the will.' However, with regard to both feminism(s) and the social model of disability, such deconstructive analyses have avoided tackling sensitive areas. For example, within 'second wave' feminism, deconstruction of the category 'woman' was initially resisted. With regard to the social model of disability, emphasis on the social model as a unifying perspective can be seen to have obscured deconstructive analyses related to areas such as 'impairment' and 'defect'.

Binary distinctions

As highlighted in Chapter 1, it is possible to assert that until relatively recently feminism, particularly 'second wave' feminism,[3] and the social model of disability tended to rely on structural either/ or analyses. Accordingly, unitary categories such as 'woman' or 'disabled person' were repositioned, revalued and re-explored in relation to the unitary category 'man' or 'able-bodied' person. It is also apparent that binary arguments pervade the opposition of medical and social model definitions of disability. The former stresses objectivity by reference to standardised classification criteria, whilst the latter focuses on self-assessed needs and rights and the extent of the debarring factors.

Writers within the disability rights movements, such as French (1993) and Morris (1993a), critique the adoption of either/or positions with either/or implications. French, like feminist writers critiquing an oversimplifying or over-rigid definition of feminism, takes issue with similar tendencies in the disability movement. French, although a supporter of the social model of disability, believes that the 'most profound problems experienced by people with certain impairments are difficult, if not impossible, to solve by social manipulation' (French 1993: 17). She goes on to say:

> When discussing these issues with disabled people who adhere strictly to the definition of disability as 'socially imposed restriction', I am either politely reminded that I am talking about 'impairment' not 'disability', or that the problems I describe have nothing to do with my lack of sight but do indeed lie 'out there' in the physical and social environment; my lack of perception of this is put down to my prolonged socialisation as a disabled person. Being told that my definitions are wrong, that I have not quite grasped what disability is, tends to close the discussion prematurely; my experiences are compartmentalised, with someone else being the judge of which are and which are not worthy of consideration. This gives rise to feelings of estrangement and alienation.
>
> (French 1993: 19)

Morris (1993a) also implicitly critiques the adoption of either/or positions with either/or implications, such as community care (with the exploitation of female carers) versus residential care (with the imposition of dependency). In this Morris takes the discussion in relation to disabilities further than writers such as Finkelstein (1993b) for whom meanings and associations tend to remain fixed. For example, residential care would always be associated with dependency, and the possibility of different associations tends not to be explored.

Issues of unity

Largely as a result of either/or dichotomies, or an over-reliance on binary forms of analysis, disability rights movements and feminism(s) in the past have often been presented as homogeneous and unified movements, with feminism appearing to speak for all women, and disability rights movements, based on the social model of disability, appearing to speak for all disabled people. The need for unity can be seen to be related to the promotion of a particular political platform, usually one that focuses on rights and resistance to the status quo. Faith (1994) highlights how, in relation to feminism, rights-based strategies have been employed to counteract subordinate status. She does, however, point to the contradiction, which applies equally well to disability rights movements, of 'using a privileged male system of power to challenge a privileged male system of rights' (Faith 1994: 60). As Faith maintains in relation to feminism, rights-based unitary movements will inevitably result in some gains, some reversals and some failures. There will also be, as Butler (1995) highlights, inevitable contestation of the unitary nature of the movement. There can be seen to be an obvious resonance here with disability rights movements and the place of individuals with learning difficulties for example. Both Faith and Butler draw from Foucault to present arguments which have relevance for the debates in Chapter 5. However, in relation to this chapter it is pertinent to note that within feminism, challenges to the feminist 'we' came from black women, working class women and others, excluded by the prevailing descriptive content of feminism. Butler observes:

> The minute that the category of women is invoked as *describing* the constituency for which feminism speaks, an internal debate invariably begins over what the descriptive content of the term will be . . . But every time that specificity is articulated, there is resistance and factionalisation within the very constituency that is supposed to be *unified* by the articulation of its common element.
>
> (Butler 1995: 49)

The question of difference

As discussed, there are similarities between disability movements and so-called 'second wave' feminism, in that, although discussion and debate are taking place, disability movements can still be seen to place particular emphasis on a unified approach and on the maintenance of a clear political message. As a result, mixed views have been presented about the opening up of greater debate about issues relating to such areas as gender, impairment, 'race' and age, in case a focus on these dimensions leads to fragmentation. Emphasis on individual identities and experience as a means of countering the assumed homogeneity of the women's movement in the 1980s did lead to fragmentation and to the dilution of sloganising messages, but it also led to a burgeoning of debate and arguably the involvement of a greater range of women in feminist issues. Voices calling for change within disability rights movements based on the social model of disability include those of Begum (1992), who emphasises the need for feminism to actively take on board disability issues and for the social model of disability and disability rights movements to explore gender differences. Abu-Habib (1997), talking about the work of Oxfam with disabled women particularly in the Middle East, maintains:

> We soon saw that we needed to consciously reject simplistic analyses which focus on disability in isolation from other important issues and social relations. Most importantly, we recognised that disabled people are not sexless: they are men and women with different interests, different characteristics including age, economic status, aspirations and different life experiences.
>
> (Abu-Habib 1997: 11)

Morris (1993a, 1996a) similarly draws attention to the ways in which homogeneity is assumed, particularly by male members of the disability rights movement, and highlights differences between disabled people. She further criticises feminists, such as Gillian Dalley (1988), who have referred to able-bodied women as 'carers' and ungendered disabled people as those who are 'cared for'. Morris insists that disabled women and men 'care for' too and highlights interrelationships and interdependency.

Both Morris (1993a) and Begum (1992) have used the feminist slogan 'the personal is political' as a means of linking personal experiences to the political arena and highlighting gender differences. These are two areas which require further exploration. The first relates to the ways in which 'experience' has been used and the second to issues associated with disability and 'impairment'.

The place of experience

With regard to the place of 'experience', there can be seen to be similarities with 'second wave' feminism and with debates relating to antiracism. In the 1980s some feminists regarded the exploration of individual experiences as being the key to breaking down the unitary category of 'women' (Spender 1985; Stanley and Wise 1983, with revised perspective in second edition, 1993). To use feminism here as a point of critique, undoubtedly, the utilisation of individual experience to challenge oppressive structures and categorisation processes can be useful in certain sets of circumstances. However, 'experience' and the utilisation of experiential accounts, as recent feminist analyses have shown, is an area fraught with difficulty. Hollway (1989: 106) maintains that 'The idea of women's experience seems to reduce to biology through idealism. Women know by virtue of being women.'

The use of personal experience to resist an oppressive label or to challenge an oppressive construct can be seen to lead to competition about who has the most claim to mount such challenges. For example, if two disabled women, one white and one black, experience the same event differently, whose account is seen to be the most accurate? Similarly, if only disabled people can challenge disablist perspectives, is this not likely to lead to further marginalisation, rather than as Oliver (1996) advocates, full integration into society, based on citizenship rights and entitlements? The consequences of claiming legitimacy by citing validating oppressive categories, then using personal experience as a reliable guide to truth have been highlighted by Adams (1989) in relation to feminism. She asserts: 'To get our spot on the balance sheet, we spend more time trying to demonstrate our oppression than we do dismantling it' (Adams 1989: 30). It can lead to a situation where one's right to speak or challenge is related to one's personal experience of disablism. Challenging disablism then becomes the discreet province of 'the disabled'.

Kelly et al. (1994) strongly criticise arguments that seek to validate positions simply on the basis of experience. In a discussion about violence, they assert:

> One does not have to have experienced an event or a form of oppression in order to develop committed understandings . . . the specifics of our particular location in systems of oppression need not be determining of either our understanding or our practice.
> (Kelly et al. 1994: 29–31)

Gilroy (1992: 57), talking about antiracism, draws attention to the ways in which ethnicity can be used 'to wrap a spurious cloak of legitimacy around the speaker who invokes it'. Barrett (1987), when discussing difference as experiential diversity, critiques the politics of difference based on individual experience and refers to the early women's liberation project of 'consciousness raising' which she says 'was based on a recognition of the fact that each woman's experience needed to be made collective in order to be understood; that is, it needed to be theorised' (Barrett 1987: 32). Brah points to the limitations of the consciousness raising method but asserts, 'Nonetheless there was at least an implicit recognition in this mode of working that experience did not transparently reflect reality, but instead it was a constellation of mediated relationships, a site of contradictions to be addressed collectively' (Brah 1992: 141). Accordingly, Brah points to the need to re-emphasise a notion of experience, not as an unmediated guide to 'truth', 'but as a practice of making sense, both symbolically and narratively; as struggle over material conditions and over meaning' (Brah 1992: 141).

Maynard (1994) focuses on using theory as an interpretative, synthesising process which makes sense both of the experience and connects experience to understanding. She maintains that for feminism to confront racism and analyse the interrelationship between class, 'race', gender and other forms of oppression, experience has to be translated into theory and theoretical perspectives used to address gaps and silences in research and literature more generally. She says: 'It is not always necessary to include women who are white, black, working class, lesbian or disabled . . . to be able to say something about racism, classism, heterosexism and disablism' (Maynard 1994: 24).

With regard to debates surrounding the slogan 'the personal is political', feminist writers, such as Fraser (1993) and Flax (1992b), have highlighted the usefulness of making public private miseries and of viewing self-defined need as publicly actionable. They have also emphasised the importance of interdependence rather than dependence. Accordingly, they can be seen to have contributed towards turning the political slogan 'the personal is political' towards 'the private is political'; a slogan which, for the reasons outlined above, may have more utility for disability rights movements.

For nearly all writers in the disability arena, fearful of the continued imposition of able-bodied agendas and perspectives, personal experience continues to occupy a position of central importance. The costs in terms of this leading to able-bodied people being excluded from participating in and supporting disability rights campaigns tend to be overlooked, in favour of disabled people grouping together on the basis of disablist experiences and developing a communal voice to challenge and campaign for change.

Disability and 'impairment'

Debates focusing on whether impairments should be incorporated into the social model of disability or excluded are currently taking place within disability rights movements. Shakespeare (1994: 283) suggests that 'some of the lack of weight given to cultural imagery and difference stems from the neglect of impairment'. French (1993: 2) accepts that an emphasis on impairments and differences between disabled people is 'politically dangerous', but maintains that it is important to discuss all aspects of disability and interaction and to focus on areas of concern, rather than adhere to what can appear to be an over-rigid theory. She emphasises differences caused by impairments and asserts:

> Whilst I agree wholeheartedly that the social model of disability represents the most important way forward for disabled people, and I understand the forces which have shaped the definition of disability to that of social oppression, I also believe that the time has now come to broaden and intensify our examination of disability and to develop and deepen our knowledge, to the benefit of all who define themselves as disabled.
>
> (French 1993: 24)

Crow (1996) also argues for a reformulated social model which fully integrates disability with impairment. She states that there has been a tendency to centre on the social model of disability to such an extent that impairment has been presented as 'irrelevant, neutral and, sometimes, positive, but never, as the quandary it really is' (Crow 1996: 58). She argues for a redefinition of impairment away from the medically orientated 'personal tragedy' construct, towards the self-interpretation of impairment and the inclusion of this interpretation within a renewed social model of disability. She maintains that with this approach, 'the experiences and history of our impairments become a part of our autobiography. They join our experience of disability and other aspects of our lives to form a complete sense of ourselves' (Crow 1996: 61).

Oliver (1996), to counteract the criticism levelled at the social model of disability by supporters such as Crow (1996), French (1993) and Morris (1993a), creates a dichotomy between 'disablement' which he asserts 'is nothing to do with the body' but 'is a consequence of social oppression', and impairment, which he says is 'nothing less than a description of the physical body' (Oliver 1996: 35). Both Finkelstein (1993a) and Oliver (1996) maintain that the conflation of disability and 'impairment' would result in the fragmentation of the disability movement, creating hierarchical distinctions which could be used to re-establish hierarchical groupings. Oliver (1996) emphasises that the social model of disability is not a social theory and that as a model it is both liberating and practically useful in that it forces professionals to critically assess their practice and to pressurise for political change in terms of rights and citizenship entitlements. He maintains that the social model of disability can contribute to a social theory of disability which must also contain a theory of impairment. However, for the purposes of the social model of disability, he insists that impairment and disability are not the same and require the development of separate models.

However, it is possible here to draw parallels with Connell's (1985) work which focuses on theorising gender. Connell critiques the ways in which various forms of biological determinism have been socially used to 'fix' gender differences. He highlights the ease with which biological connections are used to generate self-serving arguments:

> The social categories of gender are quite unlike other categories of
> social analysis, such as class, in being firmly and visibly connected
> to biological difference and function in a biological process. It is
> therefore both tempting and easy to fall back on biological
> explanation of any gender pattern. This naturalisation of social
> processes is without question the commonest mechanism of sexual
> ideologies.
>
> (Connell 1985: 266)

Connell's insistence on the importance of distinguishing between biological and social processes, emphasising that it is social processes and issues of meaning which have to be investigated and that biological matters are at best marginal, has resonance for discussions about 'impairment' and 'disability'. Accordingly, it is argued that Oliver's concern about the message of the social model of disability being diluted and subject once more to medical discourses, if discussions about impairment are incorporated, can be seen as misplaced. Within the social model of disability, 'disability' refers to social processes and 'impairment' to biological factors, yet arguably 'impairment', although linked to biology in a comparable way to a person's sex, is also a social process with its significance being associated with the meanings prescribed. Connell asserts:

>The social is radically un-natural, and its structure can never be
>deduced from natural structures. What undergoes transformation is
>genuinely transformed. But this un-naturalness does not mean
>disconnection, a radical separation from nature. Practical negation
>involves an incorporation of what is negated into the transformed
>practice. A practical relevance is established, rather than a
>determination, between natural and social structures.
>
>(Connell 1985: 269–70)

In similar terms an argument can be made for a 'practical relevance' to be established between biology and 'impairment', and between 'impairment' and 'disability'.

Connell, in the context of developing a theory of gender, argues that such a theory, rather than being a tightly knit logical system, is a 'network of insights and arguments about connections' (Connell 1985: 261). This can be seen to have relevance for the development of a social theory of disability. Oliver maintains that the social model of disability does not constitute a social theory of disability, and this has to be accepted. It does have to be borne in mind, however, that emphasis on the social model of disability within the disability movement, with the concomitant exclusions and prohibitions, could make it extremely difficult to develop a social theory of disability which appropriately develops connections with key areas such as impairment.

Disability and the body

Discussions of the body tend to be of three main types. The first focuses on the actual corporeal body, the second on the abstracted body, and the third addresses both areas. In this section, discussion will relate to the first of these areas, with the second and third areas being explored in Chapter 5.

Feminism(s) has critiqued the objectification and also the idealisation of the body, especially in terms of how female bodies are used to market commodities and how the search for the perfect body has generated vast profits for companies exploiting this. However, as Wendell (1996) points out, although feminism(s) has examined new reproductive technologies and areas concerned both with the body and with medicine for able-bodied women, issues relating to the medicalisation of the body and control over the body for disabled women have been ignored. Accordingly, the belief that the body, which includes all bodily functions, can be controlled has not been questioned. This results in the continued legitimisation of control by others, when it becomes apparent that an individual has 'lost control' over their own body. Similarly, feminism(s) has also tended to operate on the assumption that women, once they have become aware of how their bodies are being appropriated, have the physical and mental capacity to resist. This may not always be the case for disabled women and indeed for other women, and this again remains an issue that has been under-explored.

Within feminism(s), although the literature relating to 'the body' is rapidly increasing, impairment, in terms of the strong emotions displayed by able-bodied women towards women with visibly in-complete or disabled bodies, still appears to be both an under-discussed and an under-researched area. Fears of incapacity may be the reason for such a lack of attention. Indeed it is only relat-ively recently, through campaigns mounted by organisations of disabled people, that the messages associated with images of in-complete or impaired bodies have started to convey more than total negativity and pitying abhorrence.

Bodies are not just biological, physiological entities, but sites of meaning, both positive and negative, for the individual concerned. It is the appropriation of meaning by able-bodied women and men that can be seen to cause further difficulties for disabled women and men and subject them to the negative stereotypical categor-icalism of bodily impairment, in addition to the generally embracing categoricalism of appearances.

Disability and oppression

The social model of disability clearly links disability to oppression.[4] Oliver (1990) regards 'disability' as not merely being socially con-structed, but socially created as a form of institutionalised social oppression that can be compared to institutionalised racism or sexism. Morris (1993a: 9) maintains: 'Our anger is not about having a "chip on your shoulder", our grief is not a failure to come to terms with disability. Our dissatisfaction with our lives is not a personality defect, but a sane response to the oppression we experience.'

Silvers (1995), viewing 'disability' from an American context, asserts:

> ... the dilemma for individuals with disabilities lies not in their personal differences but in how the sheer specificity of historical circumstance marginalises them socially and consequently, morally as well. It is from the latter diminution that policy makers routinely have gained permission to debar the disabled from the benefits of public programs, from participation in such public institutions as marriage, and even from presenting themselves to the public's sight.
>
> (Silvers 1995: 52)

In terms of the ways in which notions of oppression have been used within the social model of disability, it can be seen that there has been a tendency to list oppressions in order to highlight the particular positions occupied by disabled people. Oliver (1990)[5] and Begum *et al.* (1994), for example, use the term 'double oppression' to refer to the experience of being black and disabled. Begum (1992) uses the term 'triple oppression' to refer to being female, black and disabled. Begum states: 'The triple oppression of being a black disabled woman has not been overlooked. There are profound implications for those of us who experience the oppression of racism, sexism and handicapism' (Begum 1992: 2).

This listing process can be regarded as double-edged. Such a list can serve as a useful point of reference for the individual concerned, or it could be seen as a means of administratively categorising an individual on the basis of stereotypical assumptions. The overall effect could be a focus for challenge, or it could be perceived as the imposition of an additional burden, with an individual being overwhelmed by the weight of their oppressions and rendered passive.

Graham (1997) asserts that the enumeration of oppressions is too simplistic and fails to consider how these might be interconnected in people's lives. With regard to 'race', Gilroy (1992) criticises the ways in which groups have united around a view of 'race' that focuses exclusively on a reductionist view of culture and ethnic identity. Like Graham, he is critical of how such perspectives ignore how 'race' intersects with other forms of oppression in people's lives. He is also critical of how antiracism has 'trivialised the rich complexity of black life by reducing it to nothing more than a response to racism' (Gilroy 1992: 60). These concerns are also applicable to notions of 'double' or 'triple oppression' used in relation to disability. In particular the use of reductionist labels makes it far too easy to devalue the rich complexity of the lives of disabled people and reduce such complexity to nothing more than a victim's response to disablism.

There are also interesting parallels here with feminism(s). Faith (1994) acknowledges that privileging the victim was an unintended consequence of the early outcomes of 'second wave feminism' and points out that the publicity generated and the public outcry in relation to violence against women, increased the perception of woman as powerless. Women, whilst no longer objectified as male property, became objectified as 'the victim', with the victim characterisation conflicting with demands for equality. Faith asks how those who need special protection because they are unable to defend themselves in the 'real' world, can be equal. She states that by enshrining male dominance in law, economy, science, medicine, religion and social policy, most Western societies have specifically facilitated and created rationales for female victimisation. Accordingly, 'females are reduced to their sex and to a class-based feminine gender standard which tyrannises females' (Faith 1994: 60). Hearn and Parkin (1993) draw attention to the ways in which people 'within and as social categories' are often constructed as 'a/the problem/issue' (Hearn and Parkin 1993: 156–8). They maintain that this then avoids discussion of who are the oppressors and the dominant assumptions related to able-bodiedness and mobility go unchallenged. Overall, it can be argued that the listing of oppressions can serve to objectify the disabled person, rendering challenge and resistance to such a status more difficult.

Finkelstein (1993b: 9) maintains that each form of discrimination has its 'own unique characteristics'. He makes a distinction between the oppression of disability and oppressions related to 'race' and gender. He maintains that the emphasis on 'normality' and upon physical and also behavioural interventions for disabled people has no parallel in relation to other types of oppression. He argues:

> Regarding 'race' and gender therefore, physical intervention
> like surgery on individuals could never be a route to the end of
> discrimination against these groups. This argument does not seem
> to apply equally well to the removal of discrimination against people
> who have an impairment of body or function.
>
> (Finkelstein 1993b: 9–10)

Finkelstein can be seen to have a point here, but he overlooks the varying ways (with some of these relating to physical violence) that various groupings have been encouraged/coerced to subscribe to normative frameworks. Shakespeare (1996, 1999) believes that links can be made between oppressions, but maintains that there are more points of overlap between disability and sexuality than between 'disability' and 'race' and gender. He points to the absence of role models within the family and immediate community and highlights that in relation to both disability and homosexuality, there is the need to reject the burdens of isolation and difference. Shakespeare argues that by resisting the negative implications of medical model frameworks and by focusing on the exclusion and injustice associated with disability, the disabled person can 'come out'. Shakespeare's analysis is extremely pertinent. However, it can be said that the ideology of the social model applied to self-categorising processes linked to identity formation can slide over aspects which do not fit. Similarly, complex identifications and conceptions of 'self' can be disregarded in favour of an analysis which interprets in accordance with ideology. To expand this point further, Shakespeare (1994, 1996, 1999), Silvers (1995), Wendell (1996) and Morris (1993a, 1996a), amongst many other writers in the field of disability, highlight how processes of socialisation and categorisation can result in disabled people acquiring a negative self-image. Shakespeare argues that the experience of disability as a negative identity occurs in the context of social relations which focus exclusively on 'impairment'. This, he maintains, leads to a limited number of responses being made available to the individual, all of which have negative connotations for processes of self-categorisation, views of self and identity formation. These aspects of a negative identity include the internalisation of grief and loss, of disabled people emphasising 'normality' and denying 'disability', and of using a disabled role as a means of eliciting sympathy, attention and interaction with professionals.

However, although it is possible to be critical of Shakespeare's (1996) analysis of identity formation in the way that he links his analysis of negative identity formation to social model/medical model(s) binaries, a key point that he is making is that a move away from 'medical model' scenarios enables and encourages disabled people to develop different and diverse narratives. This is important, although, as highlighted in a discussion of oppression, the denial of a positive identity to disabled people who do not embrace social model perspectives, has to be questioned.

As discussed, linearly framed understandings of oppressions can be seen to have inherent problems. There is, however, the notion of 'simultaneous oppression' to consider. Stuart (1993), in a similar manner to Finkelstein (1993a), views the oppression experienced by black people as unique. However, he critiques notions of 'double oppression' as inadequate and coins the term 'simultaneous oppression' to more accurately reflect the position of black people. He states:

> Simultaneous oppression, which I unashamedly borrow from Carby (1982), is the key to understanding the experience of black disabled people. It is a form of oppression which separates them from all other groups. I have identified three areas where I consider that black disabled people experience a distinct form of oppression. These are, first, limited or no individuality and identity; second, resource discrimination; finally, isolation within black communities and the family.
>
> (Stuart 1993: 99)

Stuart (1993) goes on to maintain that 'being a black disabled person is not a "double" experience, but a single one grounded in British racism' (Stuart 1993: 99). He uses his analysis to call for the construction of a separate and distinct identity for black disabled people.

Stuart's elucidation of 'simultaneous oppression' highlights the particular position of black disabled people. Although his conceptualisation is arguably more useful than the mere listing of oppressions, it still can be seen to retain the static victim-orientated emphasis found in terms like 'double oppression' and 'triple oppression'. Stuart does not fully address criticism that the creation of a separate and distinct identity for black disabled people could lead to further marginalisation. However, his purpose is to highlight both the usefulness of the social model of disability for black disabled people and to flag up issues of difference.

Lloyd (1995) adds significantly to this debate by drawing from black feminism and by particularly focusing on the issue of marginalisation. She says:

> ... the problems of stigma, disadvantage, oppression, identity and 'voicelessness' are compounded for people experiencing multiple discrimination. For black disabled women, for example, achieving centrality within feminist, black and disability agendas may be the way out of the trap of fragmentation, marginalisation or absorption.
>
> (Lloyd 1995: 222)

Lloyd sees black disabled women experiencing 'multiple discrimination' and she emphasises the 'simultaneity' of this discrimination. However, she positions black disabled women at the centre of campaigning movements for change and emphasises the importance of black disabled women having space to explore issues of relevance to them within the supportive frameworks of other movements. She therefore produces a model in which three concentric circles overlap, with black disabled women being positioned at the central interstices of all of the overlapping circles.

This model effectively addresses issues of marginalisation and can be seen to be useful politically in terms of black disabled women mounting an effective challenge to negative projected perceptions. However, in terms of reflecting the range of positions occupied by different people at different points in time, Williams (1992), whose work has been utilised by Lloyd, is concerned with interactions between the individual, power and society. She constructs a three-dimensional polyhedron to which she adds the axes of age, disability and sexuality to her original triangle of class, gender and 'race'. She suggests that:

> The significance of such a model is that, first, it poses a dynamic relationship between the individual, power and structure, its multifacets or many mirrors reflect the fact that social divisions impact upon people, singly or in groups in different ways, at different times, in different situations. At one or many moments, in one or many places issues of disability may be highlighted; at another moment the inequalities of class may predominate for the same person or group.
>
> (Williams 1992: 214–15)

The model emphasises that individuals are affected by different things at different times and that relationships and interrelationships are not static but frequently change. It accepts that the interaction of an individual or groups with other individuals and social structures is more involved than notions of double or triple oppression indicate. Rather than conceptualising relationships as simply being between oppressor and oppressed, the complex and dynamic interplay is highlighted. Oppression is fully recognised, but in a manner that does not deny agency.

The view put forward by Williams (1992) acknowledges that oppression has multiple and contested meanings. It also accepts differences and contradictions within categories, such as those of black, disabled, women, which have been seen to be unitary. However, lists of oppressions (e.g. Oliver 1990; Begum 1992; Begum *et al.* 1994) and to some extent orientations which focus on the interrelationships between oppressions and the importance of strategic challenge (e.g. Stuart 1993; Lloyd 1995) can be seen to assume a version of power that is top-down, imposed and viewed as an entity which people either have (and then it is measured in terms of degree) or do not have (Sawicki 1991). Perspectives which conceptualise oppressions in this way, fail to acknowledge a relational perspective that recognises that individuals from all groupings continually use and abuse power in a variety of ways in a range of different contexts. A white disabled man in a restaurant challenging its lack of facilities for disabled people, backed by a politically orientated rights-based pressure group, can appear very powerful to a black part-time waitress. In the same restaurant, the same waitress may appear powerful to a white man with learning difficulties whose eating pattern has been targeted by the waitress as potentially deterring other customers from eating there.

These arguments are not designed to deny oppressive categorisation processes, nor the effects which these can have on individuals. As Hearn and Parkin (1993) point out, the ways in which oppression or oppressions are interconnected and multifaceted has also to be fully recognised, and in a discussion of multiple oppressions and organisations they maintain that a fundamental oppression which underpins all other oppressions is that of ability. The challenge then becomes to recognise and challenge oppression, whilst fully acknowledging complexity and interrelational elements. These areas will be discussed further in Chapter 5 when the contribution which postmodern feminism(s) can make to the debate is explored.

Disability and standpoint positionings

Standpoint positions have been associated with forms of radical feminism and can be seen as giving women a particular position from which to speak. As highlighted in the section focusing on the place of experience, standpoint positions can be critiqued for relying on essentialist criteria and for inflexibility. However, Wendell (1996) maintains that a form of standpoint could be useful in the field of disability. She draws from the work of Patricia Hill Collins (1989, 1991) and her formulation of a standpoint epistemology of black feminist thought to argue for the development of a similar standpoint for disabled people. Such a standpoint would include the characteristic core themes related to the body of knowledge built up by disabled women, the varying manifestations of these core themes, and expressions of the interdependence of disabled women's experiences, consciousness and actions.

Wendell believes that, unlike some feminist standpoint epistemologies, the orientation developed by Hill Collins does not assume that similar experiences always produce similar points of view. Likewise, difference and diversity are incorporated without moving away from a key standpoint position that experience affects consciousness. This is an interesting development and one which qualifies some of the more essentialist elements to be found in feminist standpoint. However, with regard to disability, there is still the issue of marginalisation to be addressed. Shakespeare's (1996) concerns, highlighted earlier regarding the dangers associated with a slippage into identity politics, can still be seen to be valid. The privileging of experience, albeit in more nuanced ways, may also not be able to resist the bonds of inflexibility.

Nevertheless, it has to be acknowledged that increasingly leading standpoint theorists, such as Hartsock (1996), are developing flexible and plural perspectives. Hartsock (1996), for example, has moved away from emphasising a particular feminist standpoint that defines the oppression of women to focusing on situated knowledges. Situated knowledges are in turn defined as a plural conception of the truth and knowledge that facilitates the acknowledgement of multiple realities. In a similar vein profeminist men, such as Pease (1999), critique feminist standpoint theory which maintains that men and women have intrinsically different ways of knowing. In contrast, he develops a profeminist men's standpoint which emphasises reflexivity, accountability and change. Both these reformulations maintain an adherence to the importance of structural location and subjective positioning. Accordingly, where one 'stands' shapes what one can 'see' and how it is 'understood' (Pease 1999) without recourse to a fixed structural and subjective relationship to external factors and protagonists. Standpoint theory in line with such reformulations can be seen to have points of overlap with orientations drawn from postmodern feminism(s) discussed in Chapter 5 where emphasis is placed on difference, diversity and shifting positions without losing what Fraser and Nicholson (1993) refer to as the social critical power of feminism (Fawcett and Featherstone 1999).

Concluding remarks

Within this chapter it has been argued that many of the difficulties associated with 'second wave' feminism(s) are currently being experienced by disability rights movements based on the social model of disability. It has been contended that additional insights and alternative directions can be obtained by using feminism(s) and feminist analysis both as a point of comparison and as a critical tool. Accordingly, the social model of disability has been explored and critiqued in relation to areas which include deconstructive analyses, binary distinctions, issues of unity, the question of difference, the place of experience, disability and impairment, disability and the body, disability and oppression and disability and standpoint positionings.

Criticisms which have arisen from within disability rights movements based on the social model of disability have also been presented within this chapter. As discussed, these criticisms are predominantly directed towards broadening and developing the social model of disability rather than formulating new and different models. However, Wendell (1996), from an American perspective,[6] can be seen to have something additional to add in that she has drawn from feminism(s) to suggest the development of a modified standpoint position. Many of the areas discussed in this chapter will be revisited in Chapter 5 when orientations emanating from post-modern feminism(s) are considered.

Summary

- Feminism(s) has been used as a point of comparison and as a tool to constructively critique the social model of disability.

- Areas considered have included deconstructive analyses, binary distinctions, issues of unity, the question of 'difference', the place of experience, disability and 'impairment', disability and the body, disability and oppression and disability and standpoint positionings.

- It has been pointed out that there are similarities between the social model of disability and 'second wave' feminism and potential problem areas have been highlighted in accordance with the form of analysis described.

- Many of the areas discussed in this chapter will be revisited when orientations drawn from postmodern feminism(s) are considered in Chapter 5.

Notes

1 In terms of comparisons that have been made between rights-based
organisations of disabled people and black and feminist civil rights
movements, see, for example, Oliver (1983, 1996), Abberley (1987,
1997), Driedger (1989), Morris (1993a) and Finkelstein (1993a).
Shakespeare (1994) highlights the contribution made by feminist
inspired writers towards the cultural representation of impairment
(e.g. Shearer 1981; Davies *et al.* 1987).

2 A number of writers have highlighted the utility of feminist
perspectives (e.g. Begum 1992; Morris 1993a,b, 1996a; Begum *et al.*
1994; Price 1996). Stone (1984), Fine and Asch (1988), Hahn
(1988), Garland-Thompson (1994), Silvers (1994, 1995), Wendell
(1996) and Pinder (1995, 1996) have focused on gender distinctions
in relation to disability.

3 It is noted that the terms 'first' and 'second wave' feminism have
been criticised as being ethnocentric. However, the term is used here
for descriptive purposes to refer to a particular period in the history
of feminism(s).

4 It is acknowledged that definitions of oppression can vary. It is
recognised that oppression(s) is multifaceted and reflects social
divisions and power imbalances.

5 It is noted that Oliver (in Barnes *et al.* 1999) points to the difficulties
associated with the listing of oppressions.

6 It is acknowledged here that Wendell (1996), drawing from
American rather than British authors, although supporting the
political message of the social model of disability, does not see it as
being as significant as many of the other authors referred to in this
chapter.

Further reading

Begum, N., Hill, M. and Stevens, A. (eds) (1994) *Reflections: The Views
of Black Disabled People on Their Lives and Community Care*, London:
Central Council for Education and Training in Social Work, Paper
32.3.

Lloyd, M. (1995) 'Does She Boil Eggs? Towards a Feminist Model of
Disability' in Blair, M. and Holland, J. with Sheldon, S. (eds) *Identity
and Diversity: Gender and the Experience of Education*, Clevedon:
Multilingual Matters in association with the Open University Press,
pp. 211–24.

Morris, J. (1996) *Encounters with Strangers: Feminism and Disability*,
London: Women's Press.

Wendell, S. (1996) *The Rejected Body: Feminist Philosophical Reflections on Disability*, London: Routledge.

Williams, F. (1992) 'Somewhere Over the Rainbow: Universality and Diversity in Social Policy' in Manning, N. and Page, R. (eds) *Social Policy Review 4*, London: Social Policy Association, pp. 200–19.

Chapter 4

Community care: the public, the private and the interface between them

Chapter outline

In this chapter the following areas are appraised:

- notions of community, 'care' and community care
- care *in* the community
- perspectives of need
- modernising social services
- concepts of the public, the private and the interface between them

Introduction

In this chapter, public and private arenas and the interface between them will be explored in the context of communities and 'care' with regard to the issues facing women and disabled women and men. As discussed in Chapter 3, it is fully acknowledged that 'women' and 'disabled people' do not constitute unitary groupings and in this chapter these extremely broad terms will be used to make general points. Hearn (1992) emphasises that 'the public' and 'the private' are not impermeable, unbroachable categories and that there are lots of cross-overs. He also points to the different meanings that 'the public' and 'the private' can have in different analyses. These aspects have been fully taken on board. However, for the purposes of this chapter, it has proved useful to discuss paid work in relation to discussions about 'the public' arena and notions of private spaces in association with considerations of 'private' arenas. Concepts of 'community' and citizenship have been regarded as constituting the interface between 'public' and 'private' spheres and have been appraised accordingly. However, before exploring these areas, it is useful to look at the terms 'community', 'care' and 'community care' in greater detail.

'Community'

Communities can be both inclusive and exclusive. Commonalities can be shared or difference and diversity can be emphasised as key linking elements. As Pereira (1997) maintains, the word 'community' is a ubiquitous term and although it crops up in all kinds of situations, its meaning remains elusive. 'Community' is also invariably seen as a warm, persuasive and friendly word that gives the impression of inclusivity and belonging. With regard to the identification of communities, 'communities' can be formed by means of their particular geographical location. Various 'identities', related to ethnicities, sexual orientations, abilities and disabilities can also be seen or regard themselves as comprising distinct communities. In turn, there are 'communities' formed on the basis of antagonisms to other communities and communities which gain strength by struggling against oppressions.

Hirst (1994) distinguishes between communities of choice and communities of fate. Although there are exceptions, communities, defined by means of shared commonalities, can be seen to emphasise choice, whilst communities formed on the basis of difference and diversity draw attention to how communities can be constituted by communities of choice rejecting particular members. However, communities of fate, such as those formed by people from long-stay institutions being discharged into the community (Barnes 1997), can gain strength from shared experiences and shared identity and can in turn become communities of choice.

'Care'

Fiona Williams (1997) describes 'care' 'not only in terms of different contexts and relationships, but as a manifestation of different feelings and motivations: control, responsibility, obligation, altruism, love and solidarity' (Williams 1997: 81). She highlights the historical association of women with caring and emphasises the particular responsibilities which women may have in this area.

Feminists have viewed 'caring' responsibilities as falling predominantly on the shoulders of women. Undoubtedly, women comprise the majority of carers, but work by Green (1988), Fisher (1994) and Arber and Ginn (1990, 1995), amongst others, has drawn attention to the increasing number of male carers. The number of carers overall appears to be falling and available figures show a drop from 6.8 million in 1990 to 5.7 million in 1995. These changes have been attributed to changing social and demographic trends, increasing social mobility, loss of extended family and to more women working (Hurst 1999). Of the 5.7 million carers, two-thirds are identified as women and one-third men. However, differential patterns of caring between men and women have been identified, with men being more likely to be the full-time carer for their spouse, and women the full-time carers for relatives generally. It has been estimated that informal carers save the government at least £34 billion a year and current initiatives include the National Carers Strategy which also includes provision for young carers.

With regard to caring relationships, gender differences have been explored in relation to psychological well-being and quality of life factors. Research carried out by Rose and Bruce (1995) into spousal care by older people showed that male carers who had assumed heavy caring responsibilities, appeared to receive more praise and recognition for their input than women. Consequently, the male carers were generally more buoyant psychologically, more involved in carers' groups and appeared to have a better quality of life than female carers. They were also less likely to monitor their behaviour for fear of provoking a violent outburst from spouses whose condition exposed them to this risk. Female carers, on the other hand, particularly those providing assistance to those with complex needs and where the needs of the man had been privileged in the relationship, tended to have a very different outlook. Rose and Bruce (1995) say that whilst respecting differences between male carers, the very real suffering of these men and their dedicated caring, they as interviewers began to find themselves thinking of the male carers' descriptions of their caring roles in terms of a 'pet rabbit' relationship. Here the owner of the well cared for 'pet' received much admiration, praise and attention. With regard to the women, however, their husband failed to become an equivalent 'pet' and their equally conscientious care tended to be taken for granted, remained unpraised and it was far more difficult for them to take pride in it. Consequently, the impact of caring, according to Rose and Bruce (1995), appeared to have far greater impact on their quality of life and psychological well-being.

Some feminists have seen the family as reproducing forms of patriarchal relations which emphasise women's roles as carers and family servicers, and have promoted collectivist solutions for those needing 'care'. However, Morris (1993a), as highlighted in Chapter 2, has taken issue with such a limited and unidimensional view of care and carers. She highlights that disabled women care for, care about and require care, and she is critical of the ways in which feminist literature in the 1970s and early 1980s marginalised disabled women and also older women. She also highlights that a disabled woman may have to struggle with professionals to earn the right to care for her children and that notions of care and caring are far from straightforward. Graham similarly is keen to emphasise variation and she draws attention to how women occupy different positions, in terms of their access to and their responsibilities for care. She maintains that these positions can be linked to experiences of disability and also various positionings with regard to 'race', class and sexuality (Graham 1997). She also draws attention to caring relationships outside families, such as lesbian and gay relationships with regard to AIDS, and domestic service roles. She additionally highlights the difficulties faced by families split by immigration laws, who want and need to care, but are prevented from doing so.

'Community care'

Barnes (1997: 172) states that 'The concept of "care" is an inadequate one to describe what it is that needs to be delivered in order to enable people to live their lives within communities.' With regard to connecting 'community' and 'care', a number of associations have been distinguished. First there is 'care in the community', which Jones (1994) defines as professional services delivered in particular localities outside institutions. Related to this definition is the legislative context of community care provided by The Carers (Recognition and Services) Act 1995, the NHS and Community Care Act 1990, the preceding White Paper 'Caring for

People' (Department of Health 1989) and the Griffiths Report (Department of Health and Social Security 1988). In this context community care has been defined by the White Paper 'Caring for People' (Department of Health 1989), which informed the NHS and Community Care Act 1990, as: 'providing the services and support which people who are affected by problems of ageing, mental illness, mental handicap or physical or sensory disabilities need to be able to live as independently as possible in their own homes or in "homely" settings in the community' (Department of Health 1989: 3, 1.1).

Secondly, there is 'care by the community' which has been used to refer to informal care provided and organised by members of communities (Bayley 1973; Open University 1993). In this context, 'community' has largely been seen as a 'community of women'.

Thirdly, 'care for the community' has been used to refer to the structure of resources that enables communities to care (e.g. benefits, government grants to voluntary organisations, government funding of social service departments, housing benefit, etc.) (Walker 1997). Fourthly, 'care of the community' has been used to refer to formal patterns of care that are compatible with people's own cultural and class traditions and preferences (Abrams *et al.* 1989; Open University 1993).

There is obviously considerable overlap in these definitions and 'care' provided *by* or *in* the community can also be seen to require care *for* the community in terms of resources (Open University 1993). Other questions related particularly, but not exclusively, to 'care in the community' focus on who is responsible for deciding when care in the community is necessary and what type of community care is appropriate.

Symonds and Kelly (1998) draw attention to how changes have occurred in relation to how care *in* the community, care *by* the community and care *for* the community have been viewed over time. Their definitions of how these terms can be used differs from those given above. Care *in* the community, for example, is viewed as changes in the sites of care from institutions to varying types of accommodation in the community. Care *by* the community is regarded as a change in the providers of 'care', and care *for* the community relates to caring arrangements for those currently viewed as being in need of 'care'. They highlight that the only factor that has remained relatively constant over time, is the identity of the groups in receipt of care. However, even here they point to a cultural change which can be seen to have taken place in that now such groupings have a high public profile and are no longer hidden away in private or in publicly funded private places.

Overall, it can be asserted that community care means different things to different sets of people. It is not a new concept and is one that builds on definitions and conceptualisations of both 'community' and 'care'. Accordingly, it can relate to disabled women and men, formerly institutionalised, being supported (or not) to live in the community; it can refer to family members caring for/ caring about another family member at home (Morris 1993b); it can be used to signify community spirit and communities engaging in mutual support; it can be used to denote exclusions; it can also be whatever government legislation, policy documents and the concomitant interpretations define it to be.

Over the last decade a dominant interpretation of community care has focused on 'care *in* the community' as defined by Jones (1994). Before moving on to consider notions of the public, the private and the interface between them, it is useful to look at 'care in the community', the NHS and Community Care Act 1990 and at subsequent developments in greater detail.

Care *in* the community

The NHS and Community Care Act 1990 updated previous pieces of legislation (see Box 4.1) and established new procedures for arranging and paying for state-funded social care (Meredith 1995). It sought to create a new planning framework which placed emphasis on local authority social services departments working closely together with health authorities and others (such as general practitioners, family health services authorities, community health services, the Department of Social Security, housing and education authorities and voluntary bodies, etc.), to jointly agree community care plans, to commission services and to promote the mixed economy of care. In particular, via the preceding White Paper 'Caring for People' (Department of Health 1989) and accompanying guidance, a move away from 'service-led' provision towards 'needs-led' services, based on individually orientated care management systems, was advocated. The legislative guidance also emphasised separating those who assess for services from those who provide services to prevent a conflict of interest. This became known as the purchaser–provider split. The rationale for this split was based on the argument that only by separating those who assess or purchase services from

Box 4.1   The National Health Service and Community Care Act 1990

The NHS and Community Care Act 1990 updated previous pieces of legislation. Accordingly, legislation regarding community care services includes the following:

- Part of the National Assistance Act 1948: Section 29, Part III (residential care for older people) and Section 47 (if an elderly person is living in intolerable conditions or is unable to care for themselves, they can be removed to a place where they can receive care and attention).
- Section 45 of the Health Services and Public Health Act 1968 (local authorities to promote the welfare of older people).
- Section 21 of and Schedule 8 to the National Health Services Act 1977 (prevention and after care for people who are 'ill, aged and handicapped').
- Section 117 of the Mental Health Act 1983 (aftercare for people discharged from hospital who have been subject to mental health sections 3, 37, 47 and 48).
- The NHS and Community Care Act 1990 nullifies Sections 1, 2 and 3 of the Disabled Persons Act 1986 (these relate to the right for disabled people to be consulted about services; the right to make their own views known; the right to a written statement of services to be provided; the right to a written statement stipulating why services are to be discontinued; the right of appeal; and the right to nominate a representative or advocate). Section 4 of the Disabled Persons Act 1986 is emphasised (this relates broadly to the duties of the local authority under Section 2 of the Chronically Sick and Disabled Persons Act 1970, e.g. practical assistance in the home, provision of radio, television, library services, recreational, educational facilities, travelling for participation in agreed activities, the provision of holidays, meals and telephone when requested by a disabled person or their carer).
- Services under the Chronically Sick and Disabled Persons Act 1970 are not explicitly defined as 'community care' services under Section 46 of the NHS and Community Care Act 1990 but, according to Mandelstam with Schwehr (1996), there is strong evidence that they are an extension of Section 29 of the National Assistance Act 1948 and therefore can be defined as community care services. Although the subject of considerable legal dispute, it is now generally accepted that local authorities

can charge for services provided under the Chronically Sick and Disabled Persons Act 1970.
- Overall the Act makes changes to the previous legislation which facilitates and provides community care services to bring them in line with the 1990 Act. The local authority can charge for all services except those provided under Section 117 of the 1983 Mental Health Act.

those who provide and manage the services could a needs-led system for those assessed as having complex needs, be brought about.

The Conservative Government viewed local authority provided services as costly and the introduction of market forces in a mixed economy of care was justified on the basis that competition should encourage a range of providers to increase service quality and reduce prices. It was also argued that market forces would increase choice for service users, facilitate greater service user participation in planning forums and allow services to be tailored to meet individual needs. Accordingly, in the early years, local authorities had to spend 85% of their earmarked funding on stimulating growth and paying for provider services from the private and not-for-profit sectors.

Additionally, all local authorities had to implement quality assurance systems and ensure that community care plans, jointly agreed with local health authorities, were published annually and that they addressed the six key objectives highlighted by the Department of Health. The six key objectives were as follows:

- to promote the developments of domiciliary, day and respite services to enable people to live in their own homes wherever feasible and sensible;
- to ensure that service providers made practical support for carers a high priority;
- to promote a mixed economy of care;
- to make proper assessment of need and good care management the cornerstone of high quality care;
- to clarify the responsibilities of agencies to make it easier to hold them to account for performances; and
- to secure better value for tax-payers' money by introducing a funding structure for social care which ensured that all social care payments were made by local authorities on the basis of detailed assessments, rather than being provided on the basis of eligibility for income support.

The Carers (Recognition and Services) Act 1995 is linked to the NHS and Community Care Act 1990 and entitles carers to request an assessment of their own situation at the time when an assessment or re-assessment of the service user's needs is taking place. It further obliges the local authority to take into account the results of the assessment of the carer when making decisions about services to be provided to the service user. The National Carers Strategy, introduced in 1999, aims to make carers' assessments independent of service users' assessments and to make more money available to local authorities to meet carers' needs.

Care *in* the community: a critical appraisal

The legislation can be seen to have raised issues about terminology. In many respects the term 'community care' can be misleading in that the legislation and accompanying guidance refers to 'social care' rather than to 'community care'. Right-wing policy organisations such as the Institute for Economic Affairs in 1996 (Green 1996) have also sought, by means of the legislation, to portray service users and carers as 'active consumers' with regard to community care services. This emphasis on service users and carers as consumers can be seen to have been confusing in that service users and carers cannot operate as they would in a supermarket and it is a third party (i.e. the social services department) who purchases services on behalf of individuals to meet professionally identified and prioritised need. Service users cannot shop around and arguably few users have been in a position to operate as 'active consumers'. Orme (1998) comments that rather than service users and carers being able to operate as 'active consumers', the legislation and the introduction of care management has 'narrowed the focus of social work and social care practice on to individual needs which have to be assessed, codified and responded to' (Orme 1998: 615). She goes on to say that:

> Expectations that needs will be met by 'purchaser' agencies
> commissioning services from independent sector providers has
> led to the fragmentation of networks and communities, and to a
> reframing of the sector into the 'providers' competing for contracts,
> the conditions of which will be met by ungendered workers
> responding to the needs of anonymous users or customers who are

defined by their packages of care rather than by the sum total of
their experiences.

(Orme 1998: 615)

Undoubtedly, the underpinning ideology of the legislation has
been much disputed. Clarke (1996), for example, asks whether
welfare should be about an individual buying what they need using
their own resources within a targeted safety net or whether it is
about collective provision, free when needed and financed by taxation. The enactment of the NHS and Community Care Act 1990
and the directed stimulation of the private sector has additionally
raised questions about 'welfare for profit' and the commercialisation
of care. Within social services departments, means-tested charging
policies have made it clear that 'social services' are not free and the
charging of services for disabled people in receipt of incapacity
benefit has proved controversial. Similarly debates and legal challenges continue about the boundaries between free nursing care
and payment-orientated social care. Overall, to return to the original point, discussions about a benefit system for all based on
taxation (or a contributory benefits system), versus means-tested
targeted benefits for the few, still continue, although it is the latter
argument that over recent years, during both Conservative and
Labour administrations, has carried most weight.

Another aspect of the legislation and the subsequent guidance
to be considered is that both can and have been interpreted differently by different local authorities. On one level, this is appropriate in that there is great variation between the social needs of
different geographical areas, and localised responses are required.
However, on another level it has led to considerable discrepancies,
with an individual being entitled to services in one authority, but
not in another, or being charged for a service in one and not in
another, or services just not being available in one authority whilst
the same service may be widely available in another. There is also
the question of how need is interpreted. Discussion relating to how
need is to be defined and the appropriate action to be taken is
ongoing, and the work of Doyal and Gough (1991) has proved
particularly influential.

Doyal and Gough (1991) regard needs as being universally
shared and fundamental to all individuals. They maintain that the
satisfaction of basic needs such as health, autonomy, safety and
security, linked to intermediate needs (such as adequate nutri-
tion, protective housing, non-hazardous work environments, non-
hazardous physical environments, appropriate health care, security
in childhood, significant primary relationships, physical security,

economic security, safe birth control and child bearing, and a basic education) leads to the universal goal of participation. They define participation as incorporating self-determination (which includes ensuring that others are not harmed or their basic needs affected) and liberation, which is seen as full participation in a chosen form of life. They regard the ways in which these needs can be met as necessarily varying between individuals' cultures and countries, but assert that the satisfaction of need is an inalienable human right. Accordingly, they cite universal societal preconditions for need satisfaction and need optimisation. These include civil and political rights, rights of access to need satisfiers and full political participation. They maintain that human needs should take priority over other political goals. They also emphasise the importance of political negotiation with regard to ensuring that needs are addressed within policy and planning forums and highlight the important role to be played by ordinary citizens.

Doyal and Gough (1991) adopt a universalistic approach to human need, and in regarding the satisfaction of need as an inalienable human right, they highlight the importance of both bottom-up (ordinary citizens) and top-down (government, policy-makers, planners, etc.) influences. They acknowledge tensions between bottom-up and top-down approaches, but arguably do not specifically explore these in the context of specific policy initiatives. Community care can be seen to be a specific initiative which particularly highlights the tensions between top-down and bottom-up approaches to need and it is useful at this point to explore this area in more depth. Such an exploration also emphasises the opportunities and constraints posed by the NHS and Community Care Act 1990.

Box 4.2 (developed from Fawcett and Featherstone 1994) demonstrates how differing approaches to assessing need can result in differing outcomes. The constraints of the NHS and Community Care Act 1990 are clearly apparent. However, there are opportunities and these can best be highlighted by reference to Box 4.2 and relate to the possibilities for increased service user involvement in determining their own needs and in contributing to service planning processes. Differing perspectives have been set out as polarised opposites to emphasise the points being made. It is also acknowledged that many authorities and individual workers in the field of community care have focused on greatly increasing service user involvement. However, monitoring reports (e.g. SSI/NHSME 1994, 1995; SSI/Audit Commission Second Review of Social Services Department Audits 1998) have shown that in general much remains to be achieved.

Box 4.2   Perspectives of need

Individual wants versus professional/agency assessed needs

Individual approach:
- Want(s) can be defined as self-assessed need. How can choice and participation be addressed if self-assessed need is not central to the assessment process?

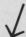

Self-assessment is seen as a central part of the assessment process.

Professional or agency approach:
- Professional or agency perspectives can view 'want' as illegitimate, potentially infinite and undeserving, and 'assessed need' as legitimate and quantifiable. The NHS and CC Act 1990 specifies the necessity of professional assessment of need despite consumer rhetoric.

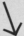

Agencies and professionals determining what constitutes need.

Service needs perceived by service users versus service needs perceived by agencies

How is policy and practice determined?

NHS and CC Act 1990 guidance insists consultation take place, but there are numerous interpretations of 'consultation'. Also highlights differences between 'empowerment' and consultation.

Philosophy/practice
'Top down'

Philosophy/practice
'Bottom up'

Need versus available resources

Tension: who is involved in determining the amount of money available, how it will be spent and accountability processes?

'Bottom up'

'Top down'

NB Both 'bottom up' and 'top down' represent extreme ends of a continuum.

Individual wants versus professional/agency assessed needs

With regard to individual wants versus professional/agency assessed needs, the tensions between professional/agency assessed needs, backed by the provisions of the NHS and Community Care Act 1990 and the desire of the service user to have their 'wants' or self-assessed needs attended to, are apparent. There has also been a mismatch between a policy emphasis on greater service user and carer involvement and what is actually laid down in Section 47 (1) of the NHS and Community Care Act 1990. The Department of Health (1990) *Policy Guide for Managers* maintained, for example, that users and carers should be enabled 'to exercise genuine choice and participation in the assessment of their care needs' (para. 3.18). The Department of Health's *Community Care Development Programme Consultation Document* (1995) also stated the aim of 'giving users and carers as much control as possible over the nature and delivery of community care services' (Department of Health 1995, para. 3.1.9). However, the NHS and Community Care Act 1990 states:

> Where it appears to a local authority that any person for whom they may provide or arrange for the provision of community care services may be in need of any such services, the authority . . . shall carry out an assessment of his [*sic*] needs for those services: and . . . having regard to the results of that assessment, shall then decide whether his needs call for the provision by them of any such services.
>
> (Section 47 (1))

With regard to disabled people, Section 47 (2) of the Act says:

> if at any time during the assessment of the needs of any person under subsection (1) (a) above it appears to a local authority that he [*sic*] is a disabled person, the authority:
> (a) shall proceed to make such a decision as to the services he requires as mentioned in Section 4 of the Disabled Persons (Service Consultation and Representation) Act without his requesting them to do so under that section; and
> (b) shall inform him that they will be doing so and of his rights under the Act.

It is clear that in relation to the NHS and Community Care Act 1990, disabled people lost the rights enshrined in Sections 1–3 of the Disabled Persons (Services, Representation and Consultation) Act 1986, which were never implemented (see Box 4.1). Although the legislation does not require a disabled person to request an assessment, the Act makes it clear that decision-making authority about the services to be provided rests with the social services department and their representatives.

Service needs perceived by service users and service needs perceived by agencies

In relation to this binary, it is useful to initially review how the service needs perceived by service users and carers have been affected by the implementation of the community care legislation. Shortly after the full implementation of the NHS and Community Care Act 1990, Baldock and Ungerson (1994) followed a sample of 32 newly disabled stroke sufferers for six months after their discharge from hospital. They found a variety of 'consumer' responses which they summarised in the following ways:

- Consumerist response: the respondents expected nothing from the state and intended to buy their own care out of their own resources, including private insurance.
- Privatist response: the respondents relied on a form of passive consumerism where their desire to do things for themselves became difficult to achieve when it became apparent that they could not meet their needs in 'off the shelf' acts of purchase. These respondents tended to have similar ideological frames of reference to the 'consumerists', but lacked the financial and personal resources to obtain what they needed.
- Welfarist response: the respondents believed in the welfare state and in their active rights as citizens to ensure that they received their entitlements in full.
- Client response: respondents passively accepted whatever came their way.

Baldock and Ungerson (1994) reported that those who could operate as active consumers outside the state system and those who adopted a welfarist approach fared best, although even these respondents experienced difficulties. However, those who relied on a privatist or a client response particularly struggled. Baldock and Ungerson stated:

> During the first six months home they slowly and painfully
> learned how the new, pluralist home care system worked and
> that many things would not happen unless they organised them.
> However, a lot of time passed as they gradually came to understand
> the degree to which the policy of user-led care meant they were on
> their own.
>
> (Baldock and Ungerson 1994: 186)

This rather bleak scenario has found a resonance in other research which has focused on how services can be made more responsive to the diverse needs of service users. Despite the positive focus, such research has also indicated that resource constraints, increasing prioritisation, gatekeeping requirements, various charging policies for domiciliary care and conflicts caused by purchaser–provider splits has resulted in service needs perceived by service users becoming no easier and possibly even harder to obtain (e.g. Social Services Inspectorate 1995; Godfery and Wistow 1997; Nuffield Institute for Health/Kings Fund 1998).

The above discussion emphasises problem areas and also highlights the importance of exploring further the issues relating to what is meant by service user involvement, 'consultation' and 'empowerment'.

Croft and Beresford (1992) maintain that two potentially conflicting philosophies, which come from very different directions, underpin efforts to involve people in social services. These reflect different impetuses for change which include on the one hand the growth of user movements and an associated emphasis on service user autonomy and control, and on the other a changed, marketised economy of welfare which focuses on privatisation and the notion of 'active consumers' who are consulted about general service planning and individual service packages.

Service user movements highlight the importance of self-advocacy. Here the aim is 'empowerment', where service users seek a direct say in agencies and services to gain greater control over their lives. With regard to consultation, agencies are looking for information from users to improve their efficiency, economy and effectiveness in a marketised system. These competing philosophies reflect real tensions between service agencies and service users over involvement. As Croft and Beresford (1992) point out, each is primarily concerned with meeting their own needs which are often very different.

Croft and Beresford (1992) and Beresford and Croft (1993) differentiate between consumerism or consultation, and 'empowerment'. In their view, consultation is an agency-led, top-down process which attempts to elicit service user and carer comments. 'Empowerment', on the other hand, is defined as service user and/ or carer-led initiatives to obtain autonomy, control and power.

It has, however, become apparent that 'empowerment' is a term which has been used in a variety of diverse and contradictory ways. Agencies and professionals have used it to refer to various kinds of consultative and participative processes. Disability rights groups have utilised it to refer to a collective struggle against discrimination and oppression, as a means of inextricably connecting needs with rights and challenging professional assessments of need, and as part of a campaign for effective citizenship rights enshrined in legislation. There is also debate and dispute over whether 'empowerment' is a process or an entity. Oliver (1993), for example, takes issue with those who view it as a thing that can be delivered by those who have it to those who do not. Writers such as Braye and Preston-Shoot (1995) and Ward and Mullender (1992) have also presented various ways of combining anti-oppressive and empowerment strategies. Baistow (1994) has drawn attention to how empowerment, although potentially having liberatory potential, simultaneously opens up new sorts of regulatory possibilities. She asserts that increasingly empowerment appears to be central to the continued legitimacy of welfare professionals who are choosing or being thrust into the role of 'expert empowerers'. She states:

> Far from user empowerment limiting the intervention of professionals into the lives of citizens, in current empowerment discourses we see space being created for new sorts of professional expertise to emerge and for new or transformed 'client groups' to be identified as the objects of this new type of professional attention.
>
> (Baistow 1994: 41)

Baistow similarly cites the lack of evaluation of empowering initiatives and the paradoxical silence of users' views and experiences of being empowered. She concludes by questioning whether empowerment can 'survive as objects of this new type of professional attention' (Baistow 1994: 41).

Key questions which emerge in a discussion of 'consultation' and 'empowerment' concern whether consultation is enough, and whether agencies are in a position to develop empowering strategies with service users. This latter point queries whether empowerment can be viewed as a process which professional agencies, service users and carers can jointly and actively facilitate. Dowson (1990), for example, argues that empowering processes are unlikely to be effective if responsibility rests primarily with agencies and professionals. Consequently it is asserted that movement is more likely if service user and carer groups operate as pressure groups campaigning outside agency structures for rights and finance based on citizenship entitlements. Another vital debate relates to whether it is possible for service user and/or carer groups, given different interests, needs, experiences and cultural and ethnic backgrounds, to work together to agree on courses of collective action. This latter question can be seen to be of considerable importance yet it is one that is often ignored (Fawcett and Featherstone 1996).

In order to move beyond the polarisations of 'consultation' and 'empowerment' and to actively engage service users, carers and health and social work/care workers in productive processes, Beresford and Trevillion (1995) use the term 'collaboration'. They focus on the development of collaborative skills for all participants and highlight the interrelationship between collaborative skills and a collaborative culture. There is also potential here for there to be a renewed and revised emphasis on community development. M. Barnes (1997), drawing from Doyal and Gough (1991) and their emphasis on the importance of the universal need of social participation, maintains that the objective of community care should be 'to enable those previously excluded from community to participate within it' (M. Barnes 1997: 155). This in turn would result in the transformation of communities, so that those previously excluded could move beyond the goal of basic participation to one where individuals could exercise their duties and rights as citizens.

Needs versus available resources

It has often been asserted that need is infinite, resources are not, and that rationing and prioritisation are inevitable. The amount of money to be spent on 'care in the community' is a political decision and one that is strongly influenced by the level of taxation that is regarded as acceptable to the majority of the electorate and dominant and media influenced typifications of deserving and undeserving individuals and groups. Arguably, at the macro level, by means of the democratic process in Britain, we all participate in the making of decisions about the amount of money to be made available and how it is to be used. However, at the micro level, we may not feel that we have any influence at all over how budgets

are determined, allocated and utilised. Again in terms of the polarisation depicted, there can be active involvement of service users,
social services, health workers and campaigning groups in the process, or budgetary allocation and use can be obscured on the basis
that executive control and management are required. In relation
to this latter point, M. Barnes (1997) has argued that accountability
has been affected in moves from elected to appointed executive
bodies and that performance review mechanisms, which prioritise
targets that are statistically measurable, are often inadequate.

The tensions apparent in community care policies, between a
focus on centralised budgetary allocation, executive authority,
agency determined assessments, management control of professionals, performance indicators, outputs rather than process *and*
an emphasis on the greater involvement of service users and carers
in planning both for themselves and for the locality, can be seen
to be continuing as the Labour Government introduces the 'third
way' for social services departments and the health services. It is
now pertinent to review some of these changes.

Modernising social services

The White Paper, *Modernising Social Services* (Department of Health
1998a) states:

> The last Government's devotion to privatisation of care provision
> put dogma before users' interests, and threatened a fragmentation
> of vital services. But it is also true that the near monopoly local
> authority provision that used to be a feature of social care led
> to a 'one size fits all' approach where users were expected to
> accommodate themselves to the services that existed. Our third way
> for social care moves the focus away from who provides the care,
> and places it firmly on the quality of services experienced by, and
> outcomes achieved for, individuals and their carers and families.
>
> (Department of Health 1998a: 8)

Labour's rhetoric is about 'quality' rather than needs-led services.
By means of their seven key principles,[1] they highlight their agenda
of welfare reform which broadly focuses on social inclusion by
promoting people's independence; improving the protection of
vulnerable people; and raising standards to achieve high quality
social services.

With regard to the health services, emphasis has been placed
on primary care groups becoming commissioners for services in
their areas and for such groups, health trusts and social services

departments, developing and implementing management information and performance systems that can be regularly monitored. In relation to both health and social services, nationally set objectives have to be met and locally identified targets have to be both agreed and adhered to. Set alongside these requirements, a key common objective is also 'to actively involve users and carers in planning services and in tailoring individual packages of care, and to ensure effective mechanisms are in place to handle complaints' (Department of Health 1998a: 111). The responsibility to 'involve', the form the involvement should take, and decisions about who should be involved, rest with individual agencies, but central government has placed emphasis on this area. Inevitable questions relate to whether this emphasis is sufficient and whether Labour have sufficiently addressed key issues. Beresford (1999) is critical about the absence of any reference to 'rights' in Labour's reforming directives. He maintains that the Government's advice on 'joined up thinking' is confused and asks how comfortably can user-centred social services sit with an income maintenance system tied to inadequate benefit levels, an increasing emphasis on fraud prevention, and benefit entitlement based on proving 'incapacity' and 'dependence'. There is also the thorny question of whether targets will emphasise cost-effectiveness in commissioning, rather than the tailoring services to meet individual need. Balloch (1999) comments that interagency working, intended to put users at the centre of services by cutting through bureaucratic boundaries, may serve to marginalise users and carers and make it more difficult for them to be involved in management and planning. Davies (1999) also asserts that despite the claim at the beginning of the White Paper that 'Social services are for us all' there is a continuing emphasis on targeting, means testing and charging, resulting in social services being seen as a last resort for desperate and distressed people. She says, 'rather than seeking to work in a more participatory way with diverse and marginalised user groups, services remain orientated to what professionals and their organisations judge to be in their users' best interests rather than what users say their needs are' (Davies 1999: 23).

With regard to the financing of the new initiatives, extra money is being made available. In relation to social services, this amounts to nearly £3 billion over a three-year period. However, a large proportion of this is tied to a social services modernisation fund and to the implementation of key initiatives. This has led to criticism that money available for core services and the social services infrastructure has decreased overall, and that too much is happening too fast, leading to a systems overload. The introduction of league tables and a 'naming and shaming' culture has also been regarded by many within social services departments as unhelpful (e.g. Wellard 1999; White 1999).[2] Additionally, front-line staff are feeling undervalued and a recent survey by *Community Care Magazine* (6–12 May 1999) showed that they had little respect for senior managers, felt senior managers were out of touch with what was actually going on, and believed they, as workers were under involved in new initiatives. There is also the distinct possibility of an increasing gap emerging between the Government's ambitious social policy and what social services departments can actually deliver. As with the introduction of community care legislation in 1990, social services departments may find that they are at the forefront of increased expectations and demand without the wherewithal to actually 'come up with the goods'.

Tensions between independent and voluntary organisations and central and local government also continue. Clarke (1996) highlighted how the NHS and Community Care Act 1990 and associated developments radically changed the nature of social services provision and emphasised how political commitment to the mixed economy of welfare led to independent agencies being brought into new relationships and regulations of partnership with state agencies, thus increasing parameters of dependence and control. With regard to voluntary organisations in particular this can be seen to have reduced their potential for active campaigning and for criticising policies which they view as detrimental to service users and carers.

There will continue to be variations in how different social services departments interpret guidance and the extent to which they involve service users and carers. Tensions between top-down management information systems and statistically orientated performance indicators, and the greater participation of service users and carers in planning services and in assuring that emphasis is placed on self-assessed need, as well as on locally and nationally determined targets, will continue. However, divergent but simultaneously promoted policy initiatives, as discussed above in relation to perspectives of need, have the potential to constrain, but also to promote opportunities in that there is a basis to press for the recognition of concerns and to mount campaigns for associated courses of action to be taken. This is an area which will be returned to in Chapter 6 when the utility of applications drawn from postmodern feminism(s) for social care will be considered.

Overall, as highlighted, the NHS and Community Care Act 1990 and subsequent developments can be seen to have posed both opportunities and constraints (Taylor-Gooby and Lawson 1993; Fawcett and Featherstone 1994b; Titterton 1994; Sheppard 1995; Lewis and Glennerster 1996; M. Barnes 1997; Walker 1997; Means and Smith 1998; Symonds and Kelly 1998). Constraints relate to the lack of resources made available to operate 'care in the community' in line with expectations and to meet increasing demand. The lack of resources has tended to turn needs-led initiatives into resource-driven prioritisations. Nevertheless, there have been opportunities in that carers and service users (and it is recognised that the needs of carers and service users are not necessarily the same) have obtained space to gain recognition of their needs and to press for their demands to be met. The introduction of the Direct Payments Scheme,[3] although discretionary, can be seen as a major gain here. However, care in the community will continue to be beset by tensions as competing agendas continue to clash. Performance targets set both locally and nationally and measured by performance indicators and top-down definitions of 'quality' will continue to be seen as unhelpful by disability rights organisations calling for the self-determined needs of disabled people to be regarded as rights and fully addressed (Oliver 1996).

The public, the private and the interface between them

In common parlance, the home is seen as a private area. It is enclosed and it is associated with family matters. Care, both in terms of emotional and physical care, is seen to take place within the private sphere. In contrast, the public arena tends to be defined in terms of work or activities that take place outside the home. Traditionally women have been associated with the private sphere and men with the public. Feminism(s) has highlighted the ways in which, as Lister (1997) points out, the ideological construction of the public–private divide has contributed to the opposition of justice and care and to the camouflaging of men's dependence on women for care and servicing. In this section, there is an acknowledgement that the gendered nature of the divide is changing. Increasingly, greater emphasis is being placed on the interface rather than on a rigid adherence to what can be regarded as an unhelpful dichotomy. This is not to imply that gendered distinctions have ceased to exist, or that changes have resulted in singularly positive developments for women and disabled women and men. Rather, emphasis is placed on reviewing changes in relation to 'private' and 'public' arenas and on exploring issues at the interface.

The private: roles and relationships

Disabled women and men are so often relegated to the private sphere and emphasis placed on their 'care' needs rather than upon how they view themselves and how they want to shape their future. 'Medical model' scenarios and the perpetration of a 'sick role' for disabled people, where compliance is rewarded by the social acceptance of the removal of responsibilities (Borsay 1997), can be seen to have contributed towards such privatisation.

As highlighted earlier, traditionally femininity and disability have been seen to reinforce each other and to be associated with the private sphere, whilst masculinity and disability have been seen to conflict with each other, with masculinity having a public focus and disability a private emphasis. The various feminism(s) have taken issue with notions of femininity imposed upon women, but, as discussed in Chapter 3, the position of disabled women has often been disregarded, leaving this diverse grouping especially vulnerable. With passivity and weakness (Begum 1992) perceived as key characteristics, disabled women have had to fight hard either to operate in accordance with gendered stereotypes or to contest these. Many of these contestations have been carried out in the private sphere, but increasingly disabled women are strongly articulating critiques both of femininity and of those feminism(s) that have ignored the ways in which they have been positioned. Accordingly, taken-for-granted perspectives related to disabled women and sexuality, self-image and bodily representations have been both deconstructed and reformulated. With regard to sexuality, for example, disabled women have drawn attention to how their sexual needs have been trivialised, whilst those of disabled men have been highlighted. They also focus on disabled women's vulnerability to rape and sexual abuse and how attitudes such as 'who would want to have sex with her' and 'she ought to be grateful for what she can get' have contributed towards oppression, stigmatisation, exploitation and domination.

Disabled women's and men's conceptions of what it is to be a woman or a man will vary according to degrees of discursive acceptance and challenge, circumstances, context and idiosyncratic factors. However, studies have been carried out which, although wary of additionally categorising disabled people, have identified patterns in terms of the ways in which the respondents relate to their gender. One study carried out by Gerschick and Miller (1995), focusing on disabled men's conceptions of masculinity, found that although none of the men interviewed constructed their masculinity in exactly the same way, there were three patterns that could be identified. The first of these was 'reformulation', which related to the men's redefinition of masculinity in their own terms. An example here is that of a man who views control and self-reliance as key masculine qualities. Accordingly, even though he requires physical care on a 24-hour basis, he reformulates his situation to emphasise those instances when he is displaying control and self-reliance and plays down those times when other aspects feature. The second pattern identified was that of 'reliance', which refers to the adoption of certain dominant attributes of masculinity. Here there is an emphasis on a view of 'self' being integrally associated with masculine characteristics such as independence, strength, stamina, etc. Respondents relied on a particular aspect of masculinity to retain their sense of being a man and accordingly went to considerable lengths to demonstrate their abilities in this direction. The third pattern was that of 'rejection', which entailed the renunciation of masculine standards and either the creation of individually orientated principles and practices or the rejection of masculinity as being important. According to Gerschick and Miller (1995), those respondents in the latter grouping adopted the most positive approach in that there was more potential for fluidity with regard to roles and a greater possibility of interaction between the individual and the environment.

Gerschick and Miller (1995) identified minor as well as major associations and highlighted how 'reliance' could be associated with 'reformulation' for example. Differences between disabled women and between disabled women and disabled men are considerable and have to be fully attended to. However, the identification of patterns, non-rigidly applied, can be useful in that gender constraints can be identified and avenues for action explored.

The public: public faces

Disabled women and men have had to fight to move out of private spheres into the public arena and as with battles fought within feminism(s), there have been some gains and some losses. Oliver and Barnes (1998) point to how the Disablement Information and Advice Line (DIAL) was initiated by disabled activists in Derbyshire in 1976 and run by disabled volunteers. This was soon followed by other DIAL networks, and disabled people, by running the advice lines and obtaining detailed information on local issues, were able to speak authoritatively about local problems and to propose solutions. However, this clear, direct and productive move into the public sphere soon became overshadowed by concerns that able-bodied people were taking over, relegating disabled women and men to private places. Nevertheless, the success of other initiatives, such as the Grove Road Scheme, also in Derbyshire (an integrated housing scheme planned and developed by disabled people), demonstrated that women and men with 'severe' impairments, given self-determined levels of support, were able to live independently and shape communities (Oliver and Barnes 1998).

In relation to the public world of work, despite marked changes, women are not as fully represented in the workforce as men, and disabled women and men are poorly represented indeed. This can be illustrated by focusing on social services departments. In England in 1998, only 28% of senior directing staff were female, whilst 72% of the lower grade posts were held by women. In relation to ethnicity, only 4% of senior staff in England were from ethnic minorities, and field social workers, care managers and line managers from ethnic minorities comprised between 10 and 16% of the total workforce (LGMP 1998). With regard to disabled women and men, in the summer of 1997 the economic activity rate for disabled people in the United Kingdom was less than half that for non-disabled people, i.e. 40% compared with 85% (CSO 1998). In addition, disabled men receive, on average, three-quarters of the wage of non-disabled people doing the same job, and disabled women earn two-thirds the wage of disabled men (Liberty 1994; Drake 1999). An emphasis on sheltered employment and therapeutic earnings with set wages and lack of progressive opportunities has also severely depressed wage entitlements. As Drake (1999) points out, the Disabled Working Allowance, introduced to supplement the wages of disabled people working over 16 hours a week, has led to only 10,000 out of an expected 50,000 receiving this entitlement. Low take-up has been attributed to discrimination by employers, insufficient publicity and to relatively small numbers of disabled women and men fulfilling the eligibility requirements.

It is also interesting to note that in 1997 women in full-time employment in the UK worked the longest hours (over 40 hours per week) of any European Union country, and that the situation was the same for men, who worked an average of nearly 46 hours a week. The number of women working full-time in 1997 was nearly a fifth more than in 1984, whilst the number in part-time work increased by nearly a quarter. This emphasis on long working hours and full-time work is unhelpful to disabled women and men whose abilities and disabilities fluctuate during the day. Webb and Tossell (1999), drawing from figures produced by the European Union and the Disability Alliance, state that there are just over six million disabled people in the UK, with over two-thirds being over the age of 60. Approximately two-thirds of disabled people (four million disabled women and men) are living at or below the poverty line and disabled people of working age are twice as likely to be living at or below the poverty line as their non-disabled counterparts.

Employment is a far from straightforward area with regard to disabled women and men. Disability rights movements based on the social model of disability stress the importance of paid employment in terms of disabled people achieving full citizenship rights. Current government policies are orientated towards reducing the amount of money spent on benefits for disabled people. The Disability Discrimination Act 1995, although flawed, provides anti-discriminatory safeguards in the field of employment for the first time for disabled people. Different agendas are operating, but the emphasis on paid employment is clear. What is not so clear is the availability of support mechanisms to enable disabled women and men to enter the workforce and to sustain and advance their careers. There are also issues discussed earlier about choice and whether an individual's self-assessed needs would prioritise the importance of work in relation to their overall well-being.

It has been estimated that in the UK, more than 1.2 million disabled people obtain physical assistance by means of the home care service provided by social services departments (Webb and Tossell 1999). This is a service provided predominantly by women, and public caring remains a key activity for women, who, as highlighted, continue to predominate in the lower echelons of the caring professions. 'Care in the community', with the associated purchaser–provider split, the emphasis on the mixed economy of care (minus compulsory competitive tendering) and care management systems, has tended to reduce employment prospects, conditions of service and training opportunities for many women working in this area. Many women are having to fight to retain their jobs on 'new' contracts with inferior pay and conditions in privatised or 'floated off' sectors. Increased pressure on women who work as carers and tight financial constraints have also led to decreases in the amount of assistance available to women and men requiring physical care in the community and at work. In many respects, both women who work as paid carers and disabled women and men requiring physical assistance at home and at work have been particularly affected by financial and policy restraints. Research carried out by the author (Fawcett 1999b) into how disabled women and men view developments in community care, produced comments such as, 'This is what bugs me, the fact that it's supposed to be a community package, a caring package to suit individual need and the quality of life, to give you a life in fact, but it doesn't cover that.' One respondent, used to being told that there is no money to improve her services, remarked, 'You get so despondent, because at the end of the day you feel as though you're trying to get blood out of a stone.' This disabled woman had to be got out of bed at 7.00 am every morning and undressed for bed every evening at 7.30 pm because the home care staff could not attend to her any later. It is also interesting to note that none of the respondents in the study carried out by the author saw the women who worked with them as being at fault. All had great sympathy and respect for these women. It was the 'planners', 'managers' and local and central government who were seen as being responsible. A report from the Nuffield Institute for Health and the Kings Fund (1998) relating to older people, states that many public, private and independent organisations are still providing unreliable and inflexible services and failing to give older people a say in their 'care'. These findings were reinforced by the comments of the respondents in the small-scale study conducted by the author and highlight that similar difficulties are experienced by disabled people.

Many disabled women and men are unable to take up employment opportunities unless physical assistance is provided in the workplace. As a result of underfunding and the prioritisation of needs, there can be problems in terms of the availability and flexibility of public care. The introduction of Direct Payments to disabled people to arrange their own 'care' may prove helpful although, as research carried out by Ann Kestenbaum (1998) points out, many disabled people can find themselves in a benefits trap. She highlights that an income of at least £20,000 per year is required in order to fund personal care costs. Disabled people earning under this sum have to rely on support from social services departments (via Direct Payments or other means), the Independent Living Fund, or the Government's Access to Work scheme to fund their personal care costs. Access to support from social services departments and the Independent Living Fund usually requires a means test. Kestenbaum found that in many cases, obtaining a job resulted in the individual's contribution toward the cost of their care package being increased. This often made the financial gains of working appear very small indeed. There are also problems in co-ordinating personal assistance required in the home with personal assistance required in the workplace. In very few instances would a social services care package include the workplace. An additional package with different personnel funded by the Access to Work scheme would therefore be required.

Kestenbaum's (1998) research draws attention to the complexities that 'care' or personal assistance users would have to negotiate their way through in order to work. Additional research carried out by Barnes *et al.* (1998) highlights other areas where further finance and sustained action could benefit disabled women and men. They found that existing research focusing on disabled people and employment frequently does not meet either the needs of disabled people, who often have no voice in research projects, or the needs of employers, who require access to readily utilisable information. In particular they found that disabled people from minority ethnic groups, older disabled workers and young disabled people leaving school were very under-represented, both as subjects of research into employment studies and as target groups for employment projects. In relation to this latter area, they also found that employment projects and areas such as employment training and disabled people preparing for and accessing places on particular schemes were overemphasised, while enabling disabled people to sustain employment in 'real' jobs, where they would be paid the market rate, was underemphasised. Progress and promotion also featured as under-addressed areas. They found that too much emphasis was placed on disabled people needing to change, rather than upon employers and working environments providing the required adaptations.

However, the research also found that current changes in the labour market, although presenting challenges, could also offer opportunities to disabled job seekers. In particular, part-time work, teleworking, flexi hours and self-employment could be offered by employers as 'reasonable adjustments' under the Disability Discrimination Act 1995 and current training schemes could increase the level of information technology skills available to meet employers' requirements. Additionally, attention to basic adaptations within the workplace, such as changing the height of a desk, allowing rest breaks and improving lighting, were viewed as important, although the most significant area identified related to the creation of a supportive, healthy workplace that focused on meeting the needs of all members of staff.

Overall, as stated in this section, any review of work and the public arena has to acknowledge feminist criticisms of the effects of community care policies on the employment of women within social services and health in particular, and the impact of short-term contracts, privatisation and job insecurity. Disabled women and men are similarly adversely affected as employees and as service users. With regard to disabled people, policies are currently moving away from having a compensatory emphasis, where special attention is paid to the category 'the disabled' and account is being taken of anti-discriminatory campaigns mounted by disabled women and men (Drake 1999). This is undoubtedly a positive move towards full citizenship rights for disabled people, and current legislation such as the Disability Discrimination Act 1995, although problematic, can be seen to contain opportunities in relation to employment. It nevertheless has to be stated that unhelpful working practices and benefit tangles may obscure rather than highlight such opportunities and obstruct their effective realisation.

The interface: community and citizenship

Fiona Williams (1997) stated:

> it is now a common observation that the invisible thread in government reports and policy documents that ties the notion of 'community' to that of 'care' is, by and large, 'women?' . . . But what of 'community?' . . . And what does community mean for women?' . . . Community may represent the space where women can begin to define and determine their own needs and conditions for existence. At the same time it may also represent the outer limits of women's restriction to domestic duties and limited access to an independent income and way of life – where women 'know their place'.

> (Williams 1997: 34)

The use of the terms 'space' and 'place' to explore the impact of 'community' upon women and disabled women and men can be seen to be an appropriate starting point. In this context, 'space' refers to the community as the interface between public and private spheres, where private matters and concerns, such as accessing public buildings, become translated into accessibility campaigns orientated towards disabled women and men easily utilising all public facilities. In this sense, 'community' as 'space' is positive and productive. 'Place' can be used to refer to how the 'community' can become restrictive in terms of having to 'care' or 'be cared for' for example. In this context 'place' can be used as the starting point for challenge and change.

In very general terms 'the community' can be regarded as impacting differently on 'women' and upon disabled women and men. If community is defined in terms of geographical area with support systems then 'women' are often seen as comprising 'the community' in terms of responsibilities and actions, with 'disabled people' being regarded as excluded and marginalised. If 'community' is defined as a community of disabled people fighting for rights-based citizenship entitlements, then it is non-disabled people who can be seen to be marginalised. However, as highlighted in Chapter 3, 'women' and 'disabled people' do not comprise unitary groupings and the impact of community, however defined, will vary enormously in terms of 'space' and 'place'.

Citizenship can be seen as a concept that incorporates both 'space' and 'place' in that it can be used to challenge restrictive and discriminatory notions of 'place', whilst at the same time opening up 'space' to explore tensions and opportunities. However, 'citizenship' is a popular term which has been used in very different ways by women and men and governments of all political persuasions. It has been used to denote civic virtue, responsibilities and rights, and to exclude as well as include. Lister (1997: 3) writes: 'Behind the cloak of gender-neutrality that embraces the idea (of citizenship) there lurks in much of the literature a definitely male citizen and it is his interests and concerns that have traditionally dictated the agenda.'

With regard to disability, Oliver's (1996) view of citizenship has been outlined in Chapter 2. As discussed there, he uses the work of T. H. Marshall (1952) to emphasise the lack of citizenship rights afforded to disabled people. In order to redress this imbalance, he calls for the collective empowerment of disabled people as active citizens and maintains that 'Empowered groups whose rights and responsibilities are constantly denied by a non-responsive formal political system, may seek to develop informal and more direct forms of political expression and activity' (Oliver 1996: 147).

Oliver is predominantly concerned with the rights of citizenship, which includes the right to gainful employment. He also acknowledges that the responsibilities and duties of citizenship are relevant to collective empowerment and to disabled people operating fully as citizens. However, the constitution of these responsibilities and duties is not clearly defined. In this there is a tension: if duties and obligations are taken to refer to paid employment amongst other things, so that paid employment constitutes a responsibility as well as a right, then there is a danger (particularly given current welfare reforms) of full citizenship rights being linked to gainful employment in the public sphere (Lister 1993; Department of Health 1998b). In this context, M. Barnes (1997) maintains:

> The prioritisation of paid employment over all other roles
> as a means through which citizenship can be expressed and
> experienced denies the value of other types of contributions
> and itself excludes those for whom work is not, or is no longer,
> an option.
>
> (M. Barnes 1997: 169)

In relation to issues of citizenship and community care, Orme (1998) focuses on how little attention is paid to issues of gender. She argues that by linking considerations of gender to concepts of involved citizenship, such as that advocated by Lister (1997), it is possible to move away from 'the deconstruction of users of community care into fragmented identities to which there can only be a partial response'. Similarly, the universalising of experience 'into categories of care needs which deny individuality' can also be avoided (Orme 1998: 621).

As mentioned previously, citizenship can be seen as a means of positively reconciling the public and the private, whilst at the same time emphasising 'space' and relegating 'place'. Lister's (1997) work on citizenship highlights gendered assumptions and she formulates a re-appropriation of citizenship that fully acknowledges the effects of structural constraints on women, whilst at the same time emphasising women's individual agency, linked to critical autonomy. She views citizenship as a dynamic process, which carries with it elements related to 'status' which incorporates rights and outcomes, and 'practice' viewed as a process, which includes both obligations and political participation. However, in this latter

context, Lister (1997) is keen to point out that a feminist interpretation would not make political participation an obligation as
this would create a measuring rod of citizenship against which many
women and disabled women and men would fall short because of
the constraints they have to contend with. Emphasis is therefore
placed on members of marginalised groups 'having the right and
opportunity to participate as political citizens' (Lister 1998: 72).

Lister considers the exclusionary nature of citizenship, both in
a global context in relation to the exclusions of nation states with
regard to immigrants and asylum seekers, and in a national context
with regard to how women, and it can be added, disabled women
and men, are excluded. She argues on the basis of citizenship,
viewed both as a status and a practice, for the strengths of both
universalistic arguments (on which the concept of citizenship is
premised) and those arguments which acknowledge and flag
up differences between members of excluded groupings, to be
creatively combined by means of the concept of differentiated
universalism.

Lister looks at ways of responding to difference and diversity
that do not involve qualifying and locating the rights and responsibilities of citizenship in a hierarchical framework. In this, she
constructs a threefold approach. First, definitions of political action
and civic virtue are expanded to include informal and non-
standardised forms; secondly, emphasis is placed on 'women in
their diversity as equals'; and thirdly, she proposes a 're-articulation'
of the relationship between formal and informal politics, so that
both are equally valued and influential (Lister 1997: 166).

Lister highlights the tensions particularly pertinent for women
between private caring and public earning and maintains that social
citizenship rights should be associated with a 'gendered template'
where time to care is fully taken account of in the 'synchronisation'
of employment and care (Lister 1997: 202). She calls for the development of a 'feminist citizenship praxis' (Lister 1997: 199), which
is related to a 'politics of solidarity in difference' that is pluralist,
inclusive, multilayered and which fully acknowledges the synchronisation of public and private matters.

Lister's (1997) analysis can be seen to be of considerable relevance for disabled women and men wanting full citizenship rights
in the twenty-first century. By placing emphasis on what can be
seen to be the interface between public and private spheres, she
makes it clear that in the arena of public and social policy, citizenship rights cannot straightforwardly and simply be linked to

employment status. This is important for women and disabled women and men. Her emphasis on agency moves away from women and disabled women and men being viewed and also viewing themselves as passive victims. Assumed unities and false universalisms, in relation to the category 'woman' and 'disabled people', are also rejected by this proactive understanding of citizenship, whilst at the same time structural constraints, which can also be experienced differently, are fully acknowledged. By means of a politics of solidarity in difference, differences are recognised and responded to, but common causes of concern, which will change and vary over time, are identified and joint action facilitated. Notions of community based on commonalities of interests which can be used to both mask and promote dominant interests and exclude marginalised groupings, such as disabled men and women, are also rejected by Lister's reconceptualisation of citizenship. She states that, 'Instead of obscuring diversity, division and difference, this conception would place them centre stage, providing an arena in which a transversal politics can be played out' (Lister 1998: 80).

With regard to the tensions between universalism and diversity, Lister (1998) argues that both areas can be productively entwined by means of a dynamic synthesis that retains universalist underpinnings and legitimisations whilst fully rising to the challenge of difference. This latter area will be returned to in Chapter 6 in relation to a consideration of the utility of orientations emanating from postmodern feminism(s) for disability rights movements based on the social model of disability.

Concluding remarks

Overall, discussions around the interface draw attention to how private matters, such as personal assistance, have a public resonance when related to working outside the home and how reformulated concepts of citizenship, such as that provided by Lister (1997, 1998), make clear links between the two arenas which have a resonance both for feminism(s) and for organisations of disabled people. In the next chapter, orientations drawn from postmodern feminism(s) will be considered. In Chapter 6, the applicability of these perspectives to disability rights movements based on the social model of disability will be reviewed. Accordingly, many of the areas considered in Chapters 2, 3 and 4 will be revisited and subjected to reappraisal. This is not to dismiss previously considered perspectives, but to ascertain whether postmodern feminism(s) has anything to add to ongoing debates in these areas.

Summary

* The different ways in which 'care', community and community care can be used have been emphasised. Tensions associated with 'care in the community' have been highlighted, particularly in relation to agency-led top-down and service user-initiated bottom-up approaches.

* Concepts of need, empowerment and citizenship have been critically appraised and the implications of differing interpretations reviewed.

* Notions of the private, the public and the interface between them have been examined in relation to gendered responses to disability, considerations of employment and disability and concepts of citizenship.

Notes

1 In the White Paper, *Modernising Social Services* (Department of Health 1998a), the three key themes are given as promoting independence, improving protection, and raising standards. Seven key principles are stated as follows:

    (i)   Care should be provided to people in a way that supports their independence and respects their dignity. People should be able to receive the care they need without their life having to be taken over by the social services system.

    (ii) Services should meet each individual's specific needs, pulling together social services, health, housing, education or any others needed. And people should have a say in what services they get and how they are delivered.

    (iii) Care services should be organised, accessed, provided and financed in a fair, open and consistent way in every part of the country.

    (iv) Children who for whatever reason need to be looked after by local authorities should get a decent start in life, with the same opportunities to make a success of their lives as any child. In particular they should be assured of a decent education.

(v) Every person – child or adult – should be safeguarded against abuse, neglect or poor treatment whilst receiving care. Where abuse does take place, the system should take firm action to put a stop to it.

(vi) People who receive social services should have an assurance that the staff they deal with are sufficiently trained and skilled for the work they are doing. And staff themselves should feel included within a framework which recognises their commitment, assures high quality training standards and oversees standards of practice.

(vii) People should be able to have confidence in their local social services, knowing that they work to clear and acceptable standards, and that if those standards are not met, action can be taken to improve things.

Throughout the White Paper there is an emphasis on welfare reform, social inclusion by promoting people's independence, improving the protection of vulnerable people and raising standards to achieve high quality social services.

Beresford (1999) says that if the rhetoric of *Modernising Social Services* is to become a reality then the following reforms must be enacted:

– the systematic and structured involvement of service users and their organisations in all areas and levels of social services decision making, operation and practice;
– the adequate and secure funding of organisations controlled by disabled people and service users;
– the central involvement of service users in the planning, provision and assessment of education and training;
– an emphasis on user-led quality standards and outcome definition and measurement;
– a proactive, outreach approach to the regulation of social care staff, which prioritises the voice, choice and credibility of service users;
– support for and the expansion of user-led initiatives in social services provision;
– specific support to ensure that the rights and needs of black people and minority ethnic communities are met;
– adoption of the social models of the disabled people's and service users' movements and the concept, philosophy and practice of independent living advocated by the disabled peoples movement (*Community Care Magazine* 11–17 March 1999).

2 The plethora of initiatives introduced since the Labour Party took power in May 1997 include the following (*Community Care Magazine* 6–12 May 1999):

Quality Protects
National Carers Strategy

Review of Mental Health Act 1983
Royal Commission on Long Term Care of the Elderly
Social Services White Paper Modernising Social Services 1998
Better Government for Older People Programme
National Service Frameworks
National Priorities Guidance
Crime and Disorder Act 1998
Welfare Reform Bill
Comprehensive Spending Review
Disability Rights Commission
Sex Offenders Register
Primary Care Groups
Health Action Zones
Education Action Zones
Tackling Drugs to Build a Better Britain
Family and Parenting Institute
Sure Start Programme
Social Exclusion Unit
National Childcare Strategy
Training Organisation for the Personal Social Services
Best Value Proposals under Local Government Bill
Acheson Report on Poverty and Health
Welfare to Work Programmes for Claimants
New Deal for Communities Regeneration Programme
Early Years Development Plans

3 The Community Care Direct Payments Act 1996 came into force on 1 April 1997. It enables social services departments to make cash payments to disabled people. The making of cash payments is a discretionary activity.

Further reading

Bornat, J., Johnson, J., Pereira, C., Pilgrim, D. and Williams, F. (eds) (1997) *Community Care: A Reader*, second edition, Basingstoke: Open University Press/Macmillan.

Lister, R. (1997) *Citizenship: Feminist Perspectives*, Basingstoke: Macmillan.

Means, R. and Smith, R. (1998) *Community Care: Policy and Practice*, revised edition, Basingstoke: Macmillan.

Symonds, A. and Kelly, A. (eds) (1998) *The Social Construction of Community Care*, Basingstoke: Macmillan.

Chapter 5

Postmodern feminism(s): exploring tensions, making links

Chapter outline

In this chapter the following areas are considered:

- understandings of poststructuralism and postmodernism
- links between poststructuralism and postmodernism
- feminist critiques of postmodern orientations
- similarities and differences between feminism(s) and postmodernism
- an overview of postmodern feminism
- postmodern feminism and power/knowledge frameworks
- postmodern feminism and notions of subjectivity
- postmodern feminism and matters of difference
- postmodern feminism and conceptualisations of able-bodiedness, disabled-bodiedness and the body

Introduction

This chapter explores what is meant by both poststructuralism and postmodernism and looks at how orientations derived from postmodern feminism(s) can be used to critically appraise aspects of modernism and postmodernism and to explore tensions and make links between the perspectives.[1] In order to facilitate this discussion, the relationship between poststructuralism and postmodernism will be reviewed and the ways in which the terms have been used will be explored. With regard to an exploration of poststructuralism, the work of Foucault in particular will be appraised. Feminist critiques of postmodern conceptualisations and similarities and differences between feminism(s) and postmodern feminism(s) will then be examined before moving on to a consideration of how tensions can be explored and links made between modernism and postmodernism by utilising orientations emanating from postmodern feminism(s). Possible applications of postmodern feminism(s) will then be considered in relation to power and knowledge frameworks, notions of subjectivity, matters of difference and conceptualisations of able-bodiedness, disabled-bodiedness and the body. With regard to the application of postmodern feminism(s), many of the issues raised in Chapter 2 will be subject to re-appraisal. The application of orientations derived from postmodern feminism(s) to the field of disability is appraised in Chapter 6.

Poststructuralism has been linked to postmodernism and although there are those who disagree (e.g. Huyssen 1990; Butler 1995), many authors see poststructuralism as forming part of the matrix of postmodern theory (e.g. Best and Kellner 1991; Barrett 1992; Sarup 1993). Accordingly, for the purposes of this chapter and for the book as a whole, the term 'postmodern' will be used to refer to both poststructural and postmodern perspectives. However, it is useful to start by considering the ways in which poststructuralism has influenced postmodern understandings.

Poststructuralism

Poststructuralism, as a term, has been applied to a wide range of theoretical positions (Weedon 1987) and it is useful, before moving on to consider poststructuralism, to review what is generally meant by structuralism. It has to be stated that there are a range of different meanings of structuralism. Structuralist formulations range across linguistic, developmental and economic spheres, but all can be seen to clearly refer in some way to the presence and importance of structures. By structuralism it is thus possible to refer to the application of broad nomothetic analyses which prioritise the explanatory power of linguistic, social and economic structures over individual agency and meaning.

Saussure (1974) was enormously influential in the development of modern structural linguistics. He developed the concept of language structuring meaning rather than reflecting something 'real'. He saw meanings as being socially produced and varying between different forms of discourse. According to Saussure (1974), there is a pre-given fixed structuring of language, prior to its realisation in speech or writing. He viewed language as an abstract system comprising sets of signs, each sign being made up of a signifier (sound or written image) and a signified (meaning). The connection between the two is arbitrary, rather than natural, and each sign obtains its meaning from its difference from all other signs in the language chain. However, according to Saussure, 'Although both the signified and the signifier are purely differential and negative when considered separately, their combination is a positive fact' (Saussure 1974: 120).

As far as Saussure was concerned, once signifier and signified are combined their meaning is fixed and he saw this as a product of the conventions of a 'speech community' (Saussure 1974: 14). He regarded the individual's relationship to language as largely unconscious and asserted that language is not produced by individual subjects. However, he maintained that the language that an individual acquires is made up of fixed meanings which result from an existing social contract that is applicable to all.

As Scott (1995) points out, social structuralism can be linked to the linguistic analyses of Saussure. Accordingly, similarities can be identified between the grammatical structure of speech and the 'grammar' of social interaction in that interactions and social relations can be appraised by reference to an underlying structure of social relations (Scott 1995: 155). Levi-Strauss (1949) drew on the work of Saussure and by means of his work on kinship in which he developed perspectives relating to the material structures of social relations, he inspired theorists such as Althusser to further develop the analysis within an economic and Marxist framework.

Althusser used the term 'ideological state apparatuses' to refer to the complex correlation of ideological and political forces within the economy (Althusser 1971). He maintained that ideological state apparatuses contribute to the reproduction of capitalist relations of exploitation and that language is the means by which the various ideological state apparatuses determine dominant meanings. Accordingly, individuals are governed by 'ideological state apparatuses' in the interests of the ruling class and by language in the form of 'ideology in general'. Ideology functions for the individual by 'interpellating', i.e. recruiting or transforming individuals into subjects and agents in relation to the various 'ideological state apparatuses' operating (Althusser 1971: 162–3). An individual's subjectivity is therefore constituted for them in language. An effect

of ideology is to make an individual unthinkingly accept their constituted subjectivity, perceiving themselves to be in control of their
own subjectivity and the formulation of meanings (Althusser 1971;
Weedon 1987).

More recently, Derrida (1978) questioned Saussure's logocen-
tricism and focus on speech. He rejected the idea that meaning
could ever be fixed and developed the concept of différance.
Derrida (1978) maintained that meaning could only be produced
via the ongoing juxtaposition of the signified and the signifier in
discursive contexts. This concept has influenced poststructural
perspectives, which view meanings as multiple, unstable, changing
and specifically related to historical, cultural and social situations.
Accordingly, it is not the spoken word or the written image that
creates meaning, but the way in which one word is associated with
another. So in one specific context the juxtaposition of 'disability'
and 'impairment' produces one set of meanings. In another, the
same juxtaposition of 'disability' and 'impairment' temporarily fixes
a different meaning. Accordingly, with regard to disability, 'impairment' is unhinged from essentialist underpinnings and the
meanings of both 'disability' and 'impairment' change according
to context.

The influence of Foucault

In relating concepts such as language and meaning to those of
knowledge and power, it is necessary to refer to discursive contexts
and to the work of Foucault.[2] Foucault's view of power and knowledge, although wide-ranging, conflationary (Dews 1979),[3] and
widely critiqued (e.g. Best and Kellner 1991; Brodrib 1992; Clegg
1992; Jackson 1992; Fraser 1993) has been extremely influential.
Clegg (1992) maintains:

> . . . his project is extremely 'constitutive' but unlike Lukes (1974)
> or Giddens (1984) the constitution is premised neither on
> 'agency' nor on the excluded 'structure'. Foucault seeks to show
> how relations of 'agency' and 'structure' have been constituted
> discursively, how agency is denied to some and given to others, how
> structures could be said to have determined some things and not
> others. The focus is on how certain forms of representation are
> constituted rather than upon the 'truth' or 'falsity' of the
> representations themselves.
>
> (Clegg 1992: 158)

Foucault developed a social relational model of power which
conceptualises power operating from the bottom up in a low profile

manner in everyday social relations or 'micropractices', rather than from the top down and requiring a high profile presence to enforce it. By 'social practices' he is referring to the planned, unplanned and taken-for-granted interactions of the everyday. To understand how power is operating, all 'micropractices' or everyday interactions and social relations have to be viewed in their discursive contexts (with discourses being defined as regimes pertaining to 'truth' by way of 'regimes of practice'). As a result, historically specific relationships emerge between combinations of power, language and institutional practices and the knowledge bases or modes of thought, which inform what is taken for granted. Foucault asserts:

> Power is employed and exercised through a net-like organisation. And not only do individuals circulate between its threads; they are always in the position of simultaneously undergoing and exercising this power. They are not only its inert or consenting target; they are always the elements of its articulation. In other words individuals are the vehicles of power, not its point of application.
>
> (Foucault 1980: 98)

The social relational model of power developed by Foucault (1980, 1981a,b) differs markedly from the juridico-discursive model (Sawicki 1991) which can be seen to inform liberal theories of sovereignty (where power is mainly viewed in terms of legislative authority, codified in law and accompanied by a theory of rights, the infringement of which becomes oppression) and Marxist theories (where power is located in the economy and the bourgeois-controlled state). According to the juridico-discursive model, power is regarded as being possessed by a particular group or located in a particular place. It is also regarded as being imposed in a top-down fashion and is predominantly repressive, focusing on prohibition backed by sanctions.

Foucault argued that the operation of power can only be understood by examining the power relations exercised within everyday social practices. He maintained that although institutions seem to reinforce particular power relations by sanctioning particular discourses, they are merely utilising the 'regimes of practice' already established. By a process which he termed 'genealogy' he sought to understand the conditions which made certain social practices or 'regimes of practices' (Foucault 1981b: 5) acceptable at a particular moment in time.

Overall, it can be asserted that Foucault focused on 'how' questions, concerned with how power manifested in social practices operates, rather than on 'why' questions that explore why social practices operate in particular ways. Fraser (1993) contends that Foucault 'calls too many different sorts of things power and simply leaves it at that' (Fraser 1993: 32). She maintains that he lacks normative resources and although it is important for Foucault's project that he can distinguish between different sorts of practices and forms of constraint, he is unable to do so. As a result, his view of how power operates tends to fluctuate between conceptualisations which ignore considerations of the value that can be attached to particular claims (Fraser 1993), and historical accounts of the operation of power which have a tendency to equate power with domination (L. McNay 1992; Fraser 1993). As Hearn and Parkin (1993) point out, Foucault's analysis does not consider the specific exploitations of oppression in their historical and material contexts. They maintain 'even in The History of Sexuality, we are left wondering what if anything happens (in discourse?) between gendered /sexual/sexualised subjects, say in the material experience of sexual violence' (Hearn and Parkin 1993: 160).

There is also power and power conceived as integrally containing points of resistance to consider. In relation to resistance, Foucault states:

> there are no relations of power without resistances; the latter are all the more real and effective because they are formed right at the point where relations of power are exercised; resistance to power does not have to come from elsewhere to be real, nor is it inexorably frustrated through being the compatriot of power. It exists all the more by being in the same place as power; hence like power, resistance is multiple and can be integrated into global strategies.
>
> (Foucault 1980: 142)

Foucault's writings on resistance can be seen to have been variously interpreted. Sawicki (1991) and Faith (1994), for example, focus on those aspects which emphasise that resistance is an integral part of power and that the two divergent aspects are always found together (Foucault 1983). However, Macdonell (1986) takes issue with Foucault's 'pragmatic' conceptualisation of resistance:

> The pragmatic standpoint, which places practice first and makes struggle secondary, cannot avoid giving precedence to power and locating resistance merely as a counter-effect in the networks of power. It thereby makes the historical existence of radical changes unthinkable.
>
> (Macdonell 1986: 124)

These debates are of considerable relevance for the discussion later in this chapter concerning the exploration of tensions and the making of links between modern and postmodern perspectives. Although complex and, as previously highlighted, open to a variety of interpretations and criticisms, Foucault's discussion of power, knowledge and resistance can be seen to have proved enormously influential in the development of ideas in the arena of postmodern feminism(s).

Postmodernity and postmodernism

With regard to terminology, postmodernity and postmodernism can be used interchangeably (e.g. Harvey 1989), or used to refer to different aspects (e.g. Bauman 1992; Sarup 1993; Smart 1993). In the context of this book, a way of managing the terms has been to equate concepts of postmodernity with the notion of a postmodern condition (or era) and to regard postmodernism (or postmodern perspectives) as referring to a variety of theoretical perspectives concerned in some way with the postmodern condition (Fawcett and Featherstone 1998).

In terms of the generally accepted aspects of postmodernism, as with poststructuralism, it is useful to start by considering what is meant by modernism. In relation to modernism there can be seen to be an emphasis on foundational thinking, on the feasibility of objective knowledge and criteria which can be disconnected from its historical, social and cultural context, and on the possibility of discovering the 'truth' of a situation. Scientific rationality holds sway and there is a belief in progress and in the binary domination of, for example, the mind over the body. There is an emphasis on universality and on large-scale grand narratives or macro theories which are seen to be all embracing and all encompassing. Table 5.1, produced by Bozalek (1999, unpublished), highlights the differences between Enlightenment or modernist ideas and postmodern conceptualisations.

Postmodernist thought emphasises diverse forms of individual and social identity where pluralism, contingency, variety, contradiction and ambivalence replace certainty, facts, objective positions and the polarisation of opposites. Fox (1993) maintains that within postmodernism, fragmentation, openness, multivocality and eclecticism hold sway and logocentrism, phonocentrism, ethnocentrism,

Table 5.1   Differences between Enlightenment or modernist ideas and postmodern conceptualisations

Enlightenment/modern ideas	Postmodern ideas
Universality	Partiality, local focus
Timelessness: knowledge is able to transcend time and space	Historical, spatial and cultural specificity; situatedness
Grand narratives	Discourses
Knowledge exists independently of any contingencies	Knowledge is influenced by bodily, historical and social contingencies
Rational thought and technological innovation can lead to progress for humanity	Reject progress through reason
Experience reflects reality	Authentic experience rejected, instead acts of power are performed and constructed in historical, social and cultural contexts
Unitary, stable, coherent, self-contained, authentic human subject	Fractured, unstable, fragmented diverse, contingent and constructed subject
Essentialism, essential identity and authentic force underlying truth (foundational knowledge)	Anti-essentialism; no essential 'core' natural to us (anti-foundationalist)
Body of received truth	Political pluralism
Claims to authority grounded in rational thought	No claims to authority; knowledge cannot be neutral and is intertwined with power
Standpoint epistemology which emphasises the experiences of the oppressed in creating privileged or true knowledge (as in feminism(s) or Marxism)	No transparent standpoint from which knowledge can be apprehended
Possibility of knowing the truth through a search for objective facts	Knowledge is shifting from context to context and is socially constructed and rooted in the values and interests of particular groups
Individual agency	Complex and overlapping amid criss-crossing elements, no unilinear direction, no cause; we as individuals have little say in who we are, individual motivations and

Table 5.1   (cont'd)

Enlightenment/modern ideas	Postmodern ideas
	intentions count for little, these are constructed within social reality imprinted by history
Concepts straightforwardly represent real objects in the world	Language or cultural practice is viewed as constructing rather than reflecting reality, and there is no transparent standpoint from which the 'real' can be apprehended. If there are no transcendental guarantees, no final source of knowledge which can be invoked as a trump card, then observation and experience are not regarded as valid
Language is transparent – it is just the medium through which representation occurs; correspondence between a truth claim (word) and the real (object)	Language constructs meaning; objects are therefore socially or linguistically constructed
Knowledge is based on neutral facts accumulated through non-obtrusive scientific means	Power is directly related to knowledge
Western (male) thinkers providing solutions for the world	Emphasises marginalised silent voices
Stability	Search for paradox, instability and the unknown
Truth	Multiple fiction
Binary opposites	Deconstruction of binary opposites
Authoritative theory beyond criticism or revision holds true over time	Shifts over time, context-specific

Source: Bozalek (1999).

phallocentrism and egocentrism are eschewed. With regard to knowledge, as a result of technical innovations, knowledge is no longer an end in itself, but a commodity to be sold (Lyotard 1984). Lyotard (1984) equates performativity with knowledge production and regards performativity as being linked to two elements of didactics. These are simple transmission reproduction (which includes technical, how to do it information) and extended imaginative reproduction (which includes imaginative and strategic thinking and problem solving). Lyotard does not see the two elements of reproduction as needing to be made available to everyone. In order to aid performativity, he maintains that extended imaginative reproduction needs only to be made accessible to those who direct and lead. Lyotard (1984) also views the 'social' as heterogeneous and non-totalisable. Accordingly, critical social theory which uses generalising categories such as gender, 'race', class, etc., is seen as too reductive of the complexity of social identities to be useful. Critiques of relations of domination and subordination which use these general categories are therefore seen as incompatible with the relativism of postmodernism (Sarup 1993).

As highlighted earlier, postmodernism is, by its very nature, impossible to delimit and define (Fox 1993), but the perceived implications of postmodernism for political action and social theory have, for some, proved unpalatable. Habermas (1981), for example, is deeply critical of the political implications of postmodernism, associating such views with fascism and anti-Enlightenment critiques (Dickens and Fontana 1994). Bauman (1992), whose response to postmodernism is more ambivalent, asserts with regard to social theory:

> It seems sometimes that postmodern mind is a critique caught at the moment of its ultimate triumph: a critique that finds it ever more difficult to go on being critical just because it has destroyed everything it used to be critical about; with it, off went the very urgency of being critical.
>
> (Bauman 1992: viii)

It is contended that in relation to maintaining the ability to critique and also to undertake political action, perspectives drawn from postmodern feminism(s) can be seen to have a contribution to make to the debates. However, before moving on to explore what is meant by postmodern feminism(s), it is useful to review feminist critiques of postmodern orientations and to consider the similarities and differences between feminism(s) and postmodern feminism(s).

Feminist critiques of postmodern orientations

It is argued in this book that orientations drawn from postmodern feminism(s) have relevance for current debates in the field of disability. However, within feminism(s), there are divergent views and these need to be attended to.

Meaghan Morris (1988), although constructively critical of both Foucault and Lyotard, calls Foucault 'a profoundly androcentric writer' (Morris 1988: 55) and advocates that his writings are treated with caution within feminism(s). Jackson (1992) similarly asks why feminists would want to engage with postmodern authors the majority of whom are men who continue to promulgate a masculine theoretical tradition. Di Stefano (1990) in a similar vein asks whether 'the uncertain promise of a political linkage between feminism(s) and postmodernism is worth the attendant political risks' (Di Stefano 1990: 77). She highlights that these risks include wondering whether feminism(s) without a subject and some kind of standpoint can survive and the dangers in a pluralist world of becoming 'an other among others' (Di Stefano 1990: 77). She states: 'It is as if postmodernism has returned us to the falsely innocent indifference of the very humanism to which it stands opposed; a rerun, in updated garb, of the modernist case of the incredible shrinking woman' (Di Stefano 1990: 77).

Alcoff (1988) contends that Foucault's constitution of the modern subject erodes the agency of feminism(s) and also its credibility and legitimacy. She argues that Foucault's perspective renders irrelevant both specific theoretical perspectives such as feminism(s) (and disability) and emancipatory movements, and destroys their normative base. Brodrib (1992) maintains that as it is only white men who have historically been recognised as subjects, it is somewhat suspect for this notion to be abolished just as white women and black people are also asserting their rights to be subjects. Deveaux (1994) warns against feminists uncritically utilising the ideas of Foucault and takes issue with the ways in which Foucault's conceptualisation of the subject erases women's specific experiences with power. She also highlights the inability of his approach to account for and articulate processes of empowerment (Deveaux 1994). Christian (1988) and Hartsock (1990) further question poststructuralist critiques of humanism and structuralism, particularly with regard to the relativistic implications for Third World and minority cultures in terms of their efforts to gain legitimacy for their struggles.

It has to be recognised that the political implications of rejecting 'grand theories' and the consequent embracing of accounts which emphasise relativity and provisionality are disturbing. Additionally, difficulties emerge when one moves away from notions of truth and the possibility of absolute underpinnings for theories. It then appears impossible to legitimate or justify one analysis over another. As highlighted, the implications of this for anti-oppressive theory and practice in relation to disability are that notions of oppression become relative and variable.

These critiques are acknowledged and the use of orientations drawn from postmodern feminism(s) are presented as a means of retaining the ability to weight criteria and respond to social divisions and social inequalities.

Similarities and differences between feminism(s) and postmodernism

There are similarities between developments in feminism(s) and postmodernism and it is useful to explore both points of similarity as well as points of difference. There are similarities in relation to a focus on deconstructive appraisals, particularly in relation to critiquing male eurocentric foundationalist knowledge claims. Differences emerge, however, in that such deconstructive appraisals have tended to be based on feminist foundational knowledge frameworks, and initially within 'second wave feminism' emphasis was placed on the unitary category 'woman' being juxtaposed with the unitary category 'man' (as discussed in Chapter 3). The ways in which such unitary categories were challenged by some feminists by means of an emphasis on essentialist notions of self and distinct subject identities, also runs counter to postmodern formulations. However, the challenges mounted within feminism(s) to the taking of essentialist positions can be seen to have points of overlap with postmodern orientations (Fawcett and Featherstone 1996).

Benhabib (1995) provides an interesting analysis when she makes links between the key theses of the postmodern position as outlined by Flax (1990) and feminism(s). She links the 'Death of Man' with the 'Demystification of the Male Subject of Reason' (Benhabib 1995: 18) which she associates with the ways in which Western reason has posited the notion of the universal ungendered singular subject. The feminist counterpoint to the 'Death of History' becomes the 'Engendering of Historical Narrative' (Benhabib 1995: 19), which she relates to the ways in which women have been denied their own history. Finally 'Death of Metaphysics' becomes 'Feminist Scepticism towards the Claims of Transcendent Reason'

(Benhabib 1995: 19) which critiques non-context-specific truth claims. However, although acknowledging similarities, she goes on to articulate problems in relation to these three distinct areas and to distinguish between 'strong' and 'weak' analyses (Benhabib 1995: 20). According to Benhabib, 'strong' analyses are those which are incompatible with the feminist project; 'weak' theses are those which are similar to feminist critiques and which can be utilised. Accordingly, with regard to the 'Death of Man', feminism has deconstructed to reconstruct; whereas 'strong' postmodernist positions postulate 'the death of the autonomous, self reflective subject, capable of acting on principle' (Benhabib 1995: 29). Similarly, the 'strong' analysis of the 'Death of History' rules out the narrative histories of marginalised groups, and the strong analysis of the 'Death of Metaphysics' undermines radical social criticism, women's agency and notions of 'self' and historical location. She maintains:

> Postmodernism can teach us the theoretical and political traps of why utopias and foundational thinking can go wrong, but it should not lead to a retreat from utopia altogether. For we, as women, have much to lose by giving up the utopian hope in the wholly other.
>
> (Benhabib 1995: 30)

Postmodern feminism(s): an overview

Postmodern feminism(s) cannot be viewed as a unified theoretical perspective and there are a number of authors who have variously engaged with both postmodernism and feminism(s). Perhaps the most influential are Fraser and Nicholson (1993) who argue for social criticism without the philosophy of an ahistorical, legitimating and transcendental discourse (Fraser and Nicholson 1993; Fraser 1995). In the development of what can be termed perspectives emanating from considerations of postmodernism and feminism(s) (or postmodern feminism(s), which is the term used throughout this book), Fraser and Nicholson distinguish between metanarratives, i.e. the histories of male dominance which claim a foundational grounding in a philosophy of history, and large-scale empirical narratives which are non-foundational and fallibilistic (Fraser and Nicholson 1993; Fraser 1995). Fraser (1995) maintains that although the former is incompatible with postmodernism, the latter is not. Her formulation can also be seen to occupy the middle ground between 'strong' and 'weak' analyses outlined by Benhabib (1995) and to relate to 'engaged historiography' disassociated from metanarratives. In the latter instance, these would include local histories focusing on lost traditions of female agency or resistance, the restoring of historicity to female-centred practices previously viewed as natural, histories that revalue subordinated cultures, and genealogies that denaturalise previously gendered categories such as 'production and reproduction', or that re-analyse the gendered subtexts of concepts such as 'class' (Fraser 1995). It also facilitates the mapping of patterns of gender relations over time, so that the complex arena of male dominance can continue to be subject to interrogation. This perspective permits both large narratives and small-scale local narratives, ensuring that the distorting tendencies of each are addressed. Accordingly, 'the result would be a post-modernist, pragmatic, fallibilistic mode of feminist theorizing that would retain social-critical, emancipatory force even as it eschewed philosophical foundations' (Fraser 1995: 62).

Fraser and Nicholson (1993) stress that theory associated with this perspective would be comparative rather than universalist and historically, temporally and culturally specific. Categories such as 'reproduction' and 'mothering' would either be rendered obsolete or genealogised and thereby placed in the framework of an historical narrative and subject to particular temporal and cultural contexts. Incorporated within such a theory would be the rejection of the idea of a subject of history and the replacement of a unitary notion of woman and feminine gender identity by plural and complexly constructed conceptions of social identity where gender would be regarded as one relevant strand amongst others. They assert that 'this theory would look more like a tapestry composed of threads of many different hues than one woven in a single colour' (Fraser and Nicholson 1993: 429).

In relation to postmodernism, a term which she continually questions, preferring to use the term poststructuralism, Butler (1995) critiques both 'for and against' analyses, which she regards as reintroducing binary frameworks, and analyses that are based on unitary and foundationalist premises. According to Butler, attempts to establish foundations lead invariably to contestation. Any category has to be unconstrained, even if this comes to serve anti-feminist purposes, although she maintains this risk is a product of the very foundationalism that it is supposed to protect feminism(s) against.

Butler sees poststructuralist analysis, which as far as she is concerned may or may not be a feature of postmodernism, as a means of overturning previously held givens and of opening up all areas for re-analysis. As she highlights, this can be regarded as a risky enterprise, but she counters the claims of those who perceive such deconstruction to be wholly negative, by maintaining that there is also much that can be regarded as productive. In relation to a poststructural analysis of violence and suffering, for example, she argues that via a poststructural deconstructive analysis, forms of violence can be understood as 'more pervasive, more constitutive, and more insidious than prior models have allowed us to see' (Butler 1995: 52). Butler can be seen to be saying that feminism(s) has been selective in its deconstructive projects, because of the perceived need to retain a foundation for re-appraisal. However, such foundations at best work both ways, and at worst operate against women. A full poststructural deconstructive appraisal opens all avenues and fully explores what Foucault (1981b) would term the genealogy of particular areas. Butler states:

> If there is a fear that, by no longer being able to take for granted the subject, its gender, its sex, or its materiality, feminism will founder, it might be wise to consider the political consequences of keeping in their place the very premises that have tried to secure our subordination from the start.
>
> (Butler 1995: 54)

Although there is much in Butler's analysis that is relevant for the current discussion, her total rejection of any kind of grounding can be seen to differ markedly from the formulation adopted by Fraser and Nicholson (1993) and Fraser (1995). Fraser (1995) argues that it is possible to adopt a position that is both anti-foundationalist and politically engaged, whilst at the same time grounding historiographies in contexts that are provisional where, it can also be asserted, the making of inter-contextual connections are facilitated. It is this latter perspective that is regarded as the most useful for the arguments developed in this book.

The orientations discussed here differ in many respects, but all can be used to critique Lyotard's position. Drawing from postmodern feminism(s), it is argued that it is possible to move beyond performativity and relativity and to explore tensions and make links between modernism and postmodernism without re-introducing binary pairings. Orientations drawn from postmodern feminism(s) can be seen to reject foundationalism, yet still be contextually and inter-contextually grounded, so that although there is a recognition that all accounts are open to change and none can be privileged, difference, diversity and social divisions can still be emphasised and addressed.

As part of this project, the contribution of perspectives derived from postmodern feminism(s) will now be examined in relation to four areas that can be regarded as key and which will be returned to in Chapter 6. These are power/knowledge frameworks, notions of subjectivity, matters of difference and conceptualisations of able-bodiedness, disabled-bodiedness and the body. It has to be acknowledged that all these areas are interlinked and that they have been separated to highlight the applicability of perspectives drawn from postmodern feminism(s).[4]

Postmodern feminism(s) and power/knowledge frameworks

Perspectives drawn from postmodernism and postmodern feminism(s) emphasise how knowledge is positioned and legitimated in relation to power. Postmodern feminism(s) rejects objective standpoints, universal and rationally sanctioned positionings and emphasises the importance of viewing all knowledge claims (including those of feminists and disabled people) as non-innocent, as privileged and as historically, socially and culturally located.

With regard to 'innocent' knowledge, Flax explores how certain knowledge claims have been located outside power relations, leading to the claim that such knowledge reveals 'the truth' and is 'for the good of all' (Flax 1992a: 447). She highlights that in accordance with such claims, those who act or are informed by such 'truths' also have their innocence guaranteed. 'Innocent knowledge' is seen to be based on and legitimated by universal reason. Objectivity is taken for granted and it is believed that such knowledge is also neutral and transparent. Postmodernism, as Flax points out, 'invites us to engage in a continual process of disillusionment' with such grandiose fantasies (Flax 1992a: 460).

Postmodern feminism(s) also points to the need to deconstruct 'privileged knowledge' claims. Here particular knowledge frames are legitimised and privileged and can be presented as 'objective'.[5] An example is the way in which 'medical models' were seen as the only way to both define and respond to disability. However, the social model of disability as developed by Oliver (1990, 1996), Finkelstein (1993a), Barnes (1990) and others, can also be given as an example of the operation of privileged knowledge. This model can be seen as primarily a materialist model located within a modernist framework. It can be presented as focused and incontrovertible. Aspects that do not fit are ignored and accordingly the positions of individuals with learning disabilities within the model are insufficiently explored (Stalker 1998); questions of culture, representation and meaning are obscured (Shakespeare 1994) and impairment is regarded as a separate area. Connell (1985), talking about gender, takes issue with analysts who 'constantly simplify radical politics and fragment it by seizing on one point of the structure to the exclusion of the rest' (Connell 1985: 263). Butler (1995) also maintains that part of the postmodernist project is to call into question the ways in which ' "examples" and "paradigms" serve to subordinate and erase that which they seek to explain . . . effecting a violent reduction of the field to the one piece of text' (Butler 1995: 37). These criticisms can be seen to apply to proponents of the social model of disability, particularly those such as Oliver (1996) who, as outlined in Chapter 2, insist that the complicating addition of 'impairment' would dilute the radical political arguments of the social model. Oliver (1996) disengages impairment from the social model of disability because it dilutes the political message and complicates an easily assimilated model, and because he fears that a focus on impairment will revive medically and hierarchically orientated constructions of disability. However, as pointed out in Chapter 2, 'impairment', like sex, can be understood as having a basic biological point of definition, but the meanings associated with both are social and diverse. Statements such as 'I am a man', 'I am a woman' or 'I have cerebral palsy' may well be biological statements of fact, but the meanings associated with each of these three simple statements are not straightforwardly biological and can be conceptualised in a number of ways which include the interpretative and interactive as well as the discursive.

As part of the deconstruction of privileged knowledge frameworks, orientations drawn from postmodern feminism(s) can be used to constructively deconstruct accepted 'facts' and to emphasise flexibility and inclusivity rather than rigidity and exclusivity. Such perspectives can also be used to emphasise that all knowledge produces its own gaps, omissions, contradictions and points of regulation. Deconstructive critiques that explore the relationship between public and private and the discursive manipulations that ensue are additionally emphasised.

In relation to power/knowledge frameworks, as highlighted earlier in this chapter, the work of Foucault has undoubtedly been

extremely influential. His work expresses shifts and changes from
the early methodological pieces (Foucault 1972) to specific historical studies or case studies on madness, criminality and sexuality.
McNeil (1993) uses the analogy of dancing to describe the constant
movements between feminism and Foucault in terms of convergence
and divergence. Foucault did not focus on issues relating to gender,
but his work can be seen to be useful to postmodern feminism(s)
in that it can be used as a catalyst for ideas. Some feminists, as
highlighted earlier, reject his contribution, but some both critically
and constructively use the work of Foucault to make connections
and to develop ideas (e.g. Butler 1990, 1995; Sawicki 1991; Fraser
1993; McNeil 1993; Hollway 1996). Foucault's (1972, 1979, 1981a,b)
critique of humanism, in particular, and the elucidation of the
operation of disciplinary power did serve to deconstruct categories
previously unquestioningly adhered to, and to point out ways in
which subjects internalised disciplinary techniques and surveilled
themselves. His emphasis on power as productive and upon power
relations operating at the micro level also opened up further areas
for analysis, and as Butler (1995) points out, his method of genealogy can be seen as a useful tool for deconstructing foundationalist
thinking.

In addition, writers such as Hollway (1996) have developed
Foucault's circulatory view of power to include a gendered analysis.
Accordingly, although power inheres in everyday social relations,
Hollway highlights that power does not have to circulate equally
or symmetrically and that it is possible to look at the varying ways
in which power circulates and to highlight difference.

Postmodernism (informed by poststructuralism) has emphasised
the integral association of power/knowledge claims and has fos-
tered the deconstruction of power/knowledge frameworks. Perspectives drawn from postmodern feminism(s) can be seen to have
further facilitated critiques of 'innocent' knowledge and to have
additionally contributed to the identification and constructive
deconstruction of privileged knowledge claims. In this latter respect,
orientations drawn from postmodern feminism(s) have (largely)
rejected the relativism of postmodernism and part of the critique
is built on an acknowledgement that although all those involved
in social practices have power, there is an acceptance that power/
knowledge operates differentially. Accordingly, deconstructive
appraisals are cognisant of such differentials and constructively take
these into account in analyses.

Postmodern feminism(s) and notions of subjectivity

Postmodernism emphasises fluidity, change and the absence of a defining individuality in relation to notions of subjectivity and the self. Essentialist experiential validity is rejected and there is also a focus on subjects being constructed in discourse and lacking subjective agency. However, writers who have engaged with postmodern feminism(s) have produced varying reformulations which reject modernist conceptualisations of a core self that is independent and self-referential whilst at the same time imbuing the subject with a form of agency and critical ability. Accordingly, subjects are not regarded as merely occupying discursive positions, but can be seen as both constructed and capable of construction and critique. Weedon, for example, asserts the following:

> As individuals we are not the mere objects of language but the sites of discursive struggle, a struggle which takes place in the consciousness of the individual. In the battle for subjectivity and the supremacy of particular versions of meaning of which it is part, the individual is not merely the passive site of discursive struggle. The individual who has a memory and an already discursively constituted sense of identity may resist particular interpellations or produce new versions of meaning from the conflicts and contradiction between existing discourses. Knowledge of more than one discourse and the recognition that meaning is plural allows for a measure of choice on the part of the individual and even where choice is not available, resistance is still possible.
>
> (Weedon 1987: 106)

Flax (1992b) focuses on citizenship and reworks the concept to incorporate a view of 'self' and citizenship which draws from postmodern feminism(s). Flax (1992b) employs a formulation that is critical of both a modern or Enlightenment view of 'self' and also a postmodern positioning of 'self'.[6] According to Flax (1992b), a postmodern feminist 'self' could be a social 'self' although it would eschew objective and rational groundings. It would also have to be placed in its historical, social and cultural context (Fawcett and Featherstone 1998).

Butler (1995) maintains that to deconstruct the subject is not the same as negating, dismissing or doing away with the subject, but opens up the term in a way that has not previously been considered or authorised. Butler argues that identity categories can never produce solidarity because they inevitably function as normative,

rather than descriptive categories and are, by implication, exclusionary. She argues that agency becomes possible by opening up
the meanings that can be associated with 'woman' and releasing it
from its categorical underpinnings. She states:

> In a sense, what women signify has been taken for granted for too
> long, and what has been 'fixed', as the 'referent' of the term has
> been 'fixed', normalised, immobilised, paralysed in positions of
> subordination. In effect, the signified has been conflated with the
> referent, whereby a set of meanings have been taken to inhere in
> the real nature of women themselves. To recast the referent as the
> signified, and to authorise or safeguard the category of women as a
> site of possible resignifications is to expand the possibilities of what
> it means to be a woman and in this sense to condition and enable
> an enhanced sense of agency.
>
> (Butler 1995: 5)

With regard to notions of the subject, subjectivity and agency,
orientations drawn from postmodern feminism(s) do not provide
a clear and integrated analysis. Indeed this is not the point. However, what they do is make links between modern and postmodern
perspectives which retain the critical edge and the overriding concerns of feminism(s) generally. Fraser (1995) gives a good example
of this when she states:

> Thus instead of clinging to a series of mutually reinforcing false
> antitheses, we might conceive subjectivity as endowed with critical
> capacities and as culturally constructed. . . . Finally, we might
> develop a view of collective identities as at once discursively
> constructed and complex, enabling of collective action and
> amenable to mystification, in need of deconstruction and
> reconstruction.
>
> (Fraser 1995: 71–2)

Postmodern feminism(s) and matters of difference

Fraser (1995) maintains that a key issue for feminism(s), and it
can be asserted for disability rights movements and other movements based on a critique of the *status quo*, is 'how to construct
cultures of solidarity that are not homogenising and repressive'
(Fraser 1995: 70). Fraser also draws attention to how 'difference'
can be used in a normative sense to gloss over pervasive differences
between women such as 'professional white middle class First World
women and the Third World women of colour they employ as
domestic workers' (Fraser 1995: 70). Similar 'glossing over' can be

seen in disability movements between academically able physically disabled individuals and those with learning difficulties.

It is argued that perspectives emanating from postmodern feminism(s) have a useful contribution to make to such discussions. In particular, approaches drawn from postmodern feminism(s) can be seen to deconstruct accepted categorisation processes and constructively address differences related to areas such as 'disability'. Williams (1996), for example, has deconstructed and reformulated perspectives of difference in relation to political understandings and the welfare context. Williams (1996) distinguishes between three different political understandings, which she calls diversity, difference and division. By diversity she refers to a shared collective experience, such as shared language or nationality; by difference she focuses on situations where shared collective experience which informs identity provides the basis for resisting the subordinate positioning of that identity; and by division, she points to situations where a dominant subject position forms an identity which protects a privileged position. She emphasises that these are not fixed categories. In relation to the questions posed by Fraser (1995) above, Williams (1996) explores the ways in which expressions of difference can lead to certain aspects of difference being focused on in an essentialist or fixed manner and other facets of an individual's or group's identity and areas of commonality with other individuals or groups, obscured. She maintains that it is possible to move beyond such a fixing of positions and use difference as a challenging and creative force by employing pragmatism and contingency. Accordingly, individuals and groups can hold multiple positions and at the same time temporarily freeze their differences for purposes of political or economic advantage. She maintains:

> The fragmentation of politics involves a constant freezing
> and melting and re-constituting of identity. At the same time,
> we cannot assume that commonalties (as women or among
> different groups) exist, nor can we override differences with
> false consciousness. But it is through the process of knowing,
> acknowledging and understanding the complex relations of power
> in which we all are caught and the differences they create that we
> can, from time to time, reach the commonalties we share.
>
> (F. Williams 1996: 72)

The issue of experience is also relevant here. As highlighted in Chapter 3, the reduction of difference to experiential diversity can be seen to have led to difficulties and to a form of uneasy pluralism within feminism (Barrett 1987). There are similar problems

surfacing with regard to disability rights movements based on the
social model of disability. However, Foucault's work has enabled
postmodern feminism(s) in its various forms to move away from
hierarchies, universalist perspectives and a valorising of difference
based on essentialist, experiential positions. Instead difference is
regarded as something that can be used productively and as a
means of multiplying the sources of resistance to particular forms
of domination (Sawicki 1991). Focusing on the topic of new reproductive technologies, Sawicki maintains in relation to this latter
point:

> Operating with a model of the social field as a field of struggle
> consisting of multiple centres of power confronting multiple centres
> of resistance prompts us to look for the diverse relationships that
> women occupy in relation to these technologies, and for the many
> intersecting subject positions constituting the social field.
>
> (Sawicki 1991: 87)

Sawicki's point can be seen to be similar to that of Williams (1996),
in that she argues for the use of all potential allies, 'even physicians'
(Sawicki 1991: 87), in particular political projects.

Overall, it is possible to assert at this point that perspectives
emanating from postmodern feminism(s) have relevance for debates in the arena of disability. In particular, discussions relating
to the temporary fixing of differences for political and strategic
ends, and the re-framing of the notion of experience, can be seen
to be eminently applicable.

Postmodern feminism(s) and conceptualisations of able-bodiedness, disabled-bodiedness and the body

In this section, in a move away from accepted understandings of
'disability' (discussed in the previous chapters), the term disabled-
bodiedness has been used. This not only emphasises that the focus
of this section is on 'the body', but also facilitates, in a non-binary
manner, the making of ongoing and varying links between conceptualisations of able-bodiedness and disabled-bodiedness.

There are many different ways of describing, conceptualising
and theorising the body. On a descriptive level, the body constitutes the visible representation of the individual. Its shape, size,
colour, presence, functionality and degree of physical intactness,
find a resonance in prevailing trends, attitudes and concepts of

able-bodiedness and disabled-bodiedness. These are simultaneously gendered and racialised. The ways in which an individual perceives their body will be influenced by how others view it and the ways in which an individual reacts to projected opinions. Moore (1994) maintains that we use our living bodies to give substance to the 'social distinctions and differences that underpin social relations, symbolic systems, forms of labour and quotidian intimacies' (Moore 1994: 71). Conceptualisations of able-bodiedness and disabled-bodiedness relate to frameworks which define 'the natural' or 'the normal'. In Western societies, a clear conceptual distinction is made between able-bodiedness and disabled-bodiedness and individuals are categorised in relation to a series of functionally orientated tests to be passed or failed depending on the particular point of view that prevails. In turn, normative frameworks are linked to theoretical perspectives, which can support, critique, overturn or reinstate various orientations at particular points in time.

Any exploration of disabled-bodiedness and able-bodiedness has first to contend with the plethora of questions which flow from any consideration of bodies, meanings, ableing or disabling criteria and conceptual frameworks. These include, who makes the distinction? What conceptual frameworks or perspectives are being utilised? What are the implications for individuals? What are the proactive and reactive factors? What about specificity and universality? The list continues, but these questions give an indication of some of the areas requiring consideration. Another difficulty refers to starting points. There are so many theoretical orientations to be examined and issues to consider that even such initial decisions become problematic. It is also impossible to consider such an exploration as having a beginning, a middle and an end. It is an area that is continually contested and continually in process. Accordingly, all points are linked to other points and all points can only be viewed as markers; repositories for information that is not fixed or static, but fluid and dynamic.

Given the complexities involved, it is useful to take this discussion further by considering a quotation from Grosz (1994: 143): 'There is no "natural" norm; there are only cultural forms of body, which do or do not conform to social norms. The problem is not the conformity to cultural patterns, models or even stereotypes, but which particular ones are used and with what effects.' Grosz focuses on the status of the body as a product and pertinently asks the question: whose product? This highlights socio-political and socio-cultural factors, prevailing ideologies, how these change in relation to place and time and how dominant frameworks can be challenged, overturned and reconceptualised by various groups. As discussed in Chapter 2, the challenges posed to the medical and welfare models of disability by organisations of disabled people can be given as an example. Functional, physical and physiological determinants that emphasise 'cure or care' are eschewed in favour of a social constructionist model that highlights social, cultural and agency/professional disabling processes.

The body, as a contested area, can be regarded as a fruitful point of exploration. This is not only in terms of the variety of conceptual frameworks that can be applied, but also with regard to the socio-political and cultural effects that divergent orientations have at various points in space and time. In this context, it has to be acknowledged that modernist views of the body remain influential. Here a mind/body split or dualism is emphasised, with the body regarded as an outer casing to the privileged inner self, whose subjectivity comprises a soul or defining essence. As L. McNay (1992), Hekman (1990) and Flax (1990) have pointed out, the modernist project draws from classical beliefs and posits binaries, which favour one aspect at the expense of the devalued other. Accordingly, mind dominates the body, reason dominates the emotions, culture dominates nature and masculinist dominates feminist. The strong in mind dominate the weak in body and the position of individuals with physical impairments is related primarily to sex, social position, access to resources and education. Postmodern conceptualisations of the body reject this mind/body split and in terms of postmodern feminism(s) there can be seen to be a revaluing of negatively perceived differences and an emphasis on multiple positionings related to varying terms of reference.

With regard to postmodern feminism(s), it is useful to focus on areas that can be regarded for the purposes of this thesis as key. Accordingly, two main areas will be considered. The first relates to Foucault and the conceptualisation of docile bodies, and the second appraises Grosz's (1994) exploration of Deleuze and Guattari's (1988) concept of the 'body without organs'.

Foucault conceptualised the body as the object, target and instrument of power and as a site of power/knowledge inscriptions. As has been discussed earlier in this chapter, power is seen as productive and Foucault maintains that a possible constitution of knowledge of the body uses an ensemble of military and educational disciplines. He asserts that it was on the basis of power over the body that a physiological, organic knowledge of it became possible and he focuses on power as a disciplinary force and as a form of surveillance and examines it by the process of genealogy. He states:

> The body is the inscribed surface of events (traced by language and dissolved by ideas), the locus of a dissociated self (adopting the illusion of a substantial unity), and a volume in perpetual disintegration. Genealogy, as an analysis of descent, is thus situated within the articulation of the body and history. Its task is to expose a body totally imprinted by history and the process of history's destruction of the body.
>
> (Foucault 1991: 83)

Foucault appears uninterested in the constitution, composition or the internal functioning of the body (Grosz 1994); rather he is concerned with the body as a site of power. Butler (1993), looking at the discursive limits of sex, both draws from Foucault and builds on his conceptualisation when she says that 'what constitutes the fixity of the body, its contours, its movements, will be fully material, but materiality will be rethought as the effect of power, as power's most productive effect' (Butler 1993: 2).

Foucault's arguments surrounding 'docile bodies' or self-disciplined human bodies where individuals surveil themselves, can also be seen to be linked to his discussions about bio-power where the body is 'directly involved in the political field' (Foucault 1979). As with most of his work, later discussions tended to reframe his original arguments and highlight different elements. Accordingly, the emphasis on 'docile bodies' subsequently can be seen to be subsumed in his analysis of 'regimes of practices' (Foucault 1981b). However, his work on 'docile bodies' has been of interest to feminists. Bartky (1988), for example, sees much in Foucault's work on disciplinary practices and the production of docile bodies that has implications for the production and reproduction of particular versions of femininity. However, she criticises Foucault for not differentiating between the bodily experiences of men and women. Bordo (1993), drawing from Foucault's assertion that where there is power there is also resistance (Foucault 1983), highlights that while performing as docile bodies, and she gives the example of the anorexic, our 'docility' can have consequences that can be seen as liberating or culturally transforming. A further example given by Bordo is how 'feminine' decorativeness may operate 'subversively' in professional contexts where masculinist norms are dominant. Bordo (1993) distinguishes between early feminist reactions to Foucault and those which draw from postmodernism and feminism(s). She says that whilst initially concepts such as 'discipline', 'docility', 'normalisation' and 'bio-power' were used to add to the prevailing discourse of men as oppressors and women as oppressed, postmodern feminism(s) has picked up on 'intervention', 'contestation' and 'subversion'. These terms have been used to critique oppressor/oppressed scenarios and to produce reformulations in which 'nomadic, fragmented active subjects' can confound dominant discourses and resist 'the "grip" of systemic power on the body' (Bordo 1993: 193–4).

However, Bordo (1993), drawing from hooks (1991), asserts that subversion of dominant cultural forms happens more easily in texts than in the everyday world of human interaction. Bordo (1993) looks at the pressures placed on women to be slim, athletic, young and beautiful and highlights how such images are often portrayed as being overtly subversive, whilst covertly normative. In relation to disability this draws attention to the ongoing obstacles associated with challenging normative discourses and in positively reframing disability as 'embodied difference' (Wendell 1996: 584).

Deleuze and Guattari (1988) also move away from modernist mind/body dualisms by foregrounding a concept of 'desire' as productive, expansionist and as a means of making links. They can be seen to distance themselves from the ambiguities inherent in Foucault's writings, with regard to the passivity of the body and the possibility of resistance, by emphasising activity in terms of the ongoing struggles between discipline and resistance to discipline (Fox 1993). Deleuze and Guattari developed the concept of a body without organs (BwO) as a way of representing the body as a broiling surface of discursive inscriptions, the body's own will to power and the positive investments of libido by others in the body. Grosz (1994) reviews the utility of the concept of the 'body without organs' from a perspective that can be seen to draw from postmodern feminism(s) and there is much in her analysis that has applicability for discussions in relation to disability. In particular, the BwO focuses on all bodies and their varying inscriptions, rather than differentiating between able-bodiedness and disabled-bodiedness.

Deleuze and Guattari see the 'body without organs' as a body composed of, and open to, all the flows and intensities of the 'desiring machines' that compose it. The BwO is conceptualised as a surface of speeds and intensities prior to being stratified, unified, organised and hierarchised. The BwO is not uniform and one differs from another in terms of movement, the flow of intensities that it produces on its surface or which it allows to be produced and the types of circulation. The emphasis is therefore not on what the BwO is and how it is composed, but on its actions, effects, functions and productive capacity. The BwO, whilst being neither a place, a plane or a fantasy, is a field for the production, circulation and intensification of desire, a focal point for the 'desiring machines' of which it is constituted.

Deleuze and Guattari's work is complex and although rejecting ideologies and macro narratives, they can be seen to produce a conceptual framework which appears no less embracing and self-referring for its coherence than modernist contributors such as Marx and Freud. They could also be accused of deterritorialising women's bodies and subjectivities only to reterritorialise them as part of their own project which could be seen to have universalist tendencies (Grosz 1994). In addition, the emphasis on forces and flows in the body (and bodies) could be seen as shifting the debate away from notions of the subject to such an extent that conceptualisations of subjectivity drawn from postmodern feminism(s) (relating to a subject being both constructed and capable of construction and critique) no longer become possible. With regard to matters of difference, there is also the charge that by eradicating notions of difference, they are merely positing a male-orientated hegemonic sameness that differs little from malestream modernist accounts. However, although there are problem areas, there can be seen to be aspects of this conceptualisation that have relevance for postmodern feminism(s) and these are discussed below.

Initially, it has to be asserted that a perspective which conceives of the body as a series of forces and intensities facilitates the reformulation of debates, such as those relating to disability, outside of the usual points of reference relating to medicalisation. Accordingly, questions related to these areas become not merely symptoms, products and effects of particular cultural dictates but 'forces, intensities, requiring codifications or territorialisations' which in turn exert 'their own deterritorialising and decodifying force, systems of compliance and resistance' (Grosz 1994: 180). Binary differentiations can also be seen to be rejected in favour of a 'both and' form of analysis which explores the development of binary practices in order to inform reformulations. Accordingly, although the utility of binary practices can be explored in terms of highlighting the operation of enduring, negative and oppressive facets of power, discussions can creatively explore similarities and the re-interpretation of aspects which relate to both sides of the binary (and in this context issues of impairment could be considered).

Prohibitions, with regard to those areas viewed as unacceptable by particular binary formulations (e.g. the ways in which operating as a 'tragic cripple' can produce responses that are unacceptable to proponents of the social model, but which the individual concerned may not want to forgo), are also opened up for discussion. Finally, the reformulation of 'desire' as a positive and productive force common to all bodies can be seen to move the discussion away from perspectives which position women and disabled people as passive objects.[7]

These discussions relating to the body have to be linked to previous debates about the contribution which perspectives emanating from postmodern feminism(s) can make to areas such as power/ knowledge frameworks, notions of subjectivity and matters of difference. As highlighted above, the contribution made by Deleuze and Guattari (1988), although not located within postmodern perspectives, can be seen to have, in relation to some of the aspects highlighted, a parallel relevance for postmodern feminism(s). A consideration of the BwO can therefore be seen to be pertinent with regard to discussions about able-bodiedness, disabled-bodiedness and the body.

Concluding remarks

In this chapter, the feasibility of using orientations emanating from postmodern feminism(s) to critically appraise aspects of modernism and postmodernism and to explore tensions and make links between modern and postmodern perspectives has been examined. The application of constructively deconstructive analyses drawn from postmodern feminism(s) to power/knowledge frameworks, notions of subjectivity, matters of difference and conceptions of able-bodiedness, disabled-bodiedness and the body, have been used to facilitate the recognition and rejection of modernist 'innocent' and 'privileged' power/knowledge claims, notions of a 'core' essentialist self, unitary undifferentiated categorisation processes and the positing of binary oppositional frameworks.

With regard to postmodern conceptualisations, critical appraisal on the basis of orientations drawn from postmodern feminism(s) has resulted in reformulations being presented. In relation to power/knowledge frameworks, the postmodern contention that it is not possible to ground power/knowledge claims has been reformulated. Accordingly, with regard to postmodern feminism(s), all power/knowledge claims are regarded as non-innocent and non-privileged, but it is seen to be possible to weight conflicting claims in particular contexts. Inter-contextual connections also become possible. With regard to notions of 'self', postmodern contentions that subjectivity is fluid and identity is not fixed have been reformulated so that emphasis is placed on the 'self' as a social entity and on the negotiation of meanings associated with interaction. In relation to difference, the postmodern emphasis on pluralism and relativity is reformulated so that it becomes possible to temporarily 'freeze' difference(s), to explore commonalities and, where agreed, to mount political campaigns for change. In turn, the ways in which bodies are inscribed has been reformulated to also take account of the capacity for agency.

Postmodernism has been criticised for focusing on the superficial and eschewing substance (e.g. Jackson 1992) or for affirming the *status quo* (Smart 1993). However, by using perspectives drawn from postmodern feminism(s), it has been argued in this chapter that it is possible to go beyond performativity and unfettered relativity and develop an approach that rejects foundationalism, yet is contextually grounded so that it remains possible to recognise and respond to social inequalities. It is also argued that this approach facilitates the development and use of theoretical tools that can be used to critically appraise aspects of modernism (which includes feminism(s) and formulations in the arena of disability) and postmodernism.[8]

Summary

- Understandings of poststructuralism and postmodernism have been appraised and, for the purposes of this book, poststructuralist understandings have been incorporated within postmodern orientations. The influence of Foucault has also been considered.

- Critiques emerging from feminism(s) of postmodern orientations have been explored and the similarities and differences between feminism(s) and postmodernism have been highlighted.

- The utility of perspectives drawn from postmodern feminism(s) as a means of exploring tensions and making links between modernism and postmodernism has been examined. It has been argued that orientations emanating from postmodern feminism(s) can be used to reject both a modernist emphasis on foundationalism and a postmodernist focus on relativity. Accordingly, although there is a recognition that change is ongoing, it remains possible to highlight factors associated with difference and diversity, whilst also continuing to recognise and respond to social divisions and particular manifestations of power.

- The contribution of perspectives derived from postmodern feminism(s) has been explored in relation to four key areas: power/knowledge frameworks; notions of subjectivity; matters of difference; and conceptualisations of able-bodiedness, disabled-bodiedness and the body.

Notes

1 As outlined in Chapter 1, it is argued that conceptualisations drawn from postmodern feminism(s) can be employed to critically appraise aspects of modernism (which can be seen to include non-postmodern versions of feminism(s) and models of disability) and postmodern perspectives.

2 The debates about whether Foucault can be regarded as a poststructuralist writer are acknowledged here (e.g. Dreyfus and Rabinow 1993).

3 Dews (1979: 165, in Clegg 1992: 208) notes Foucault's 'tendency to slide from the use of the term "power" to designate one pole of the relation power–resistance, to its use to designate the relations as a whole'.

4 Material used in this chapter has been influenced by Fawcett and Featherstone (1996, 1998) and Fawcett (1996a, 1998, 1999a,b).

5 The deconstruction of 'privileged' knowledge claims is presented in the context of feminist deconstructive appraisals. The deconstruction of 'privileged' knowledge claims have obvious points of similarity with the emphasis placed by Foucault (1972, 1979, 1981b) on the deconstruction of dominant discourses.

6 With regard to modern orientations, Flax (1992b) argues that a feminist view of an interconnected, integrated and social 'self' differs from the Enlightenment view of 'self' as unified, essential and

rational, where individuality is sovereign and inviolate. In terms of postmodern formulations, she takes issue with concepts of 'self' as a position in language propounded by Derrida (1978). Similarly, she contests Foucault's (1983) view of 'self' as an effect of discourse.

7 The work of Grosz (1994) has been influential in developing the arguments presented here.

8 It has to be stated that orientations which explore postmodern (poststructural) feminism(s) and psychoanalysis have not been utilised in this chapter (e.g. the work of Kristeva 1986; Irigaray 1993; Chodorow 1994; Cixous 1994). This relates to constraints of time and space and to an appreciation that this is a divergent subject area that would change the focus of this book. An additional point to be made here is that although such conceptualisations can be seen to have something to offer in terms of the exploration of a psyche and a sexuality that is historically and culturally specific and in the ways in which reason and a coherent sense of self give way to a notion of self that is complex and in process, there are, and in this I agree with Weedon (1987), what appear to be insurmountable problems with regard to the notion of the unconscious and the marginalisation of women within a Lacanian symbolic order.

Further reading

Bock, L. and James, S. (eds) (1992) *Beyond Equality and Difference*, London: Routledge.

Docherty, M. (ed.) (1993) *Postmodernism: A Reader*, Hemel Hempstead: Harvester Wheatsheaf.

Grosz, E. (1994) *Volatile Bodies: Towards a Corporeal Feminism*, Bloomington and Indianapolis: Indiana University Press.

Hekman, S. J. (ed.) (1996) *Feminist Interpretations of Michel Foucault*, Pennsylvania: Pennsylvania State University Press.

Nicholson, L. (ed.) (1995) *Feminist Contentions: A Philosophical Exchange*, London: Routledge.

Radtke, H. L. and Stam, H. J. (1994) *Power/Gender: Social Relations in Theory and Practice*, London: Sage.

Ramazanoğlu, C. (ed.) (1993) *Up Against Foucault: Explorations of Some Tensions Between Foucault and Feminism*, London: Routledge.

Smart, B. (1993) *Postmodernity*, London: Routledge.

Chapter 6

Postmodern feminism(s) and debates in the arena of disability

Chapter outline

This chapter will focus on the applicability of perspectives drawn from postmodern feminism to debates and discussions in the field of disability. Particular attention will be directed towards the following:

- needs, rights, citizenship and matters of difference
- privileged power/knowledge frameworks
- multiple selves
- risks, expertise and ethics
- the weighting of oppressions
- bodily considerations

Introduction

This chapter will draw from discussions contained in previous chapters to review the relevance which orientations emanating from postmodern feminism(s) can be seen to have for debates in the field of disability. As highlighted earlier, this is to proffer suggestions rather than to make definitive statements and to contribute towards debates in the field.

Needs, rights, citizenship and matters of difference

Postmodern orientations (which in this analysis incorporate post-structuralist perspectives) critique structuralist positionings. Such critiques include universalist conceptions of basic human need, such as those put forward by Doyal and Gough (1991) and discussed in Chapter 4, and notions of inalienable human rights based on fundamental citizenship entitlements. Postmodern orientations can therefore be seen to remove the very foundation of disability rights movements based on the social model of disability and to severely challenge modernist feminist movements. As highlighted in Chapter 5, just as women and disabled women and men are becoming subjects (as defined by modernism), the whole notion of the subject is being abolished.

The debate about whether we now inhabit a postmodern world or whether we are in a phase of high modernism, or a continuation of modernism, continues. However, the way in which postmodern perspectives challenge modernist emancipatory movements such as disability rights campaigns, does provide food for thought. Possible responses include the summary dismissal of such problematic perspectives, or the exploration of ways of engaging with postmodernism whilst retaining links with modernism. It is this latter project that this chapter is concerned with, and with regard to notions of needs, rights, citizenship and matters of difference, it is argued that reformulations drawn from postmodern feminism are worthy of consideration.[1]

With regard to concepts of need, reformulations derived from postmodern feminism(s) emphasise the ways in which specific needs, manifested in particular contexts, can be continually recognised in different contexts providing the basis for action. Similarly, by emphasising contextual grounding, although universalist conceptions of citizenship and rights are rejected, rights that can be weighted in particular contexts, linked to specific pieces of legislation and which facilitate inter-contextual connections, can be highlighted and fought for (Fawcett 1998). The onus is also not just on those who have direct experience of a particular aspect of discrimination to take on challenges and to press for reform, but for broad coalitions to form and reform. Such coalitions can comprise disabled-bodied and able-bodied men and women from all ethnicities, who through mediation and theorisation of their own experiences and those of others, are prepared to focus on specific issues and press for change. Issues of difference and diversity within groupings can also be attended to without the perceived need to present a particular grouping as unified and homogeneous. Accordingly, slippage into fixed identity politics, with the attendant danger of marginalisation, can be avoided.

With regard to difference, Scott (1994) maintains that 'difference' has been one of women's most creative analytical tools and one that cannot be relinquished. In contrast, Silvers (1995) argues that the legitimation of difference militates against notions of equality and inclusiveness. From a social policy context, she asserts that the formulation of social policy that reconciles equality with difference can avoid marginalisation and stigmatisation and can 'advance historically subordinated groups' (Silvers 1995: 31). She criticises 'identity' politics and cites the Americans with Disabilities Act 1990 as a piece of legislation which in the United States has neutralised 'exclusionary social practices in a way responsive to the complexities of our lives' (Silvers 1995: 52).

Flax (1992b) in turn suggests that it is necessary to go beyond linkages between equality and difference. She says that because equality as currently understood and practised is constituted confusingly, by both a denial and also a ranking of differences, it is not as useful an antidote to relations of domination as conceptualisations of justice.

As outlined in Chapter 5, Flax (1992b) connects justice to an active notion of citizenship. Citizenship can be regarded as a modernist concept, yet Flax can be seen to reformulate this notion by disassociating it from structuralist and universalist frameworks, whilst at the same time retaining a means of imbuing the term with non-essentialist features. Flax (1992b) views justice as a process and maintains that by emphasising aspects such as reconciliation, reciprocity, recognition and judgement, differences can be positively, rather than negatively valued.[2] Flax (1992b) highlights that 'justice' viewed from within this framework is not a universal concept, nor a set of finite rules; rather it is an ongoing process with varying aspects changing over time. According to Flax (1992b), this notion of 'justice' could be part of a process which facilitates the negotiation of differences between individuals and groups, without the need to either destroy or take over (Fawcett and Featherstone 1996; Fawcett 1999a).

Flax (1992b), by disassociating citizenship from universalist and structuralist roots, presents a reformulation that places responsibility for justice and citizenship on interconnected social subjects. Accordingly, there can be no recourse to foundational underpinnings: citizenship is what 'we' make it. All therefore are involved – disabled-bodied and able-bodied women and men – and citizenship evolves through social practices. Women and men are not uncritical discursively constituted subjects. They have the power to choose particular discursive subject positions and to critique.

Flax (1992b) uses the concept of citizenship in ways that are not dissimilar to Lister's reworking of the term discussed in Chapter 4. Lister (1997, 1998) makes it clear that her analysis cannot be located within a postmodern framework. However, her calls for a 'feminist citizenship praxis' (Lister 1997, 1998) which is associated with a politics of solidarity in difference and which is pluralist, inclusive and multi-layered is not that dissimilar from the concept of citizenship put forward by Flax (1992b). Lister's calls for a 'differentiated universalism' as a means of combining universalist elements of citizenship with a full consideration of the plethora of differences operating, is somewhat more at odds with conceptualisations drawn from postmodern feminism(s). However, if 'universalism' is reformulated to refer to a form of grounding that is historically, culturally and socially specific and which also takes full account of context, then Lister's analysis has considerable relevance for postmodern feminism(s) and also for reformulated notions of citizenship that could be used by disability rights groups. Put simply, citizenship, viewed in this way, can be taken to refer to inclusion in all social, political, economic and cultural activities for all those residing in a particular country at a particular point in time. Mechanisms for both identifying and addressing differences can also be clearly formulated. However, definitions of difference and exclusion, and the means of identifying and addressing these exclusions, will change over time.

Privileged power/knowledge frameworks

In relation to power/knowledge frameworks, as discussed in Chapter 5, postmodern feminism(s) can be seen to facilitate a change of orientation away from fixed notions of 'truth', towards culturally, historically and socially situated perspectives of knowledge. Knowledge claims are viewed as being integrally associated with power and power/knowledge paradigms, and are not regarded as 'innocent' or objective. There is a recognition that although all participants in any interaction utilise power, this does not lead to the assumption that power and knowledge are evenly distributed, or operate equally.

Orientations emanating from postmodern feminism(s) relating to the constructive deconstruction of prevailing power/knowledge frameworks place emphasis on the identification of privileged perspectives and on the manner in which power/knowledge frameworks operate. In relation to this last point, subjects can be positioned in particular ways by the operation of power/knowledge frameworks, or subjects can position, utilising the power/knowledge frameworks available in indirect, direct, covert or overt ways. Examples here can be taken from research engaged in by the author (Fawcett 1999b) which looked at how subjects both position and are positioned in interview accounts read as texts. All the subjects were 'registered disabled', i.e. they were regarded as being disabled by others. Interviews were carried out with 14 women and 11 men from four case-study settings. These comprised an 'innovative' residential centre where staff were employed to be the 'arms and legs' of residents, a 'traditional' residential centre, the community, and a day centre for disabled people. At the time the interviews took place, residents from both the 'innovative' and the 'traditional' residential centres were being encouraged to move out into the community by the social services departments responsible for these facilities. The majority of the residents were not in favour of such a move, fearing isolation, poor services and the lack of physical (and in some cases emotional) support.

Many of the texts from the 'innovative' residential centre and the 'traditional' residential centre contain elements which highlight that the subjects, although 'consulted' about changes taking place in relation to their centres, did not feel that their opinions carried any weight at all in decision-making processes. The social services departments can be seen to have positioned the subjects as being in need of guidance and direction, with *their* direction being clear and unquestionably right. At points in the texts, the subjects resist their positioning and position in a way that can be read as privileging alternative perspectives. The social services departments can be seen to position directly, whilst the sometimes challenging positionings of the subjects veer towards the indirect and covert. Examples are given below.

KB, from the 'innovative' residential centre, is a 57-year-old white man who severed his spine in a bicycle accident nine years ago. He says that in an ideal world there ought to be more centres like the one he is currently living in. He states, 'there are so many people that have gained in my view, gained so much benefit from this [centre], companionship and genuine care and so many options given'. In the text, the centre is contrasted negatively with 'the community' where KB says so many are 'having to fight, they're having to state their claim every time, they're having to make sure that the qualities of care don't deteriorate'. KB makes it clear that he would prefer to stay but, despite his wish to remain and concerns about living on his own in the community, he is being 'encouraged' to move out. However, KB can be seen to resist this positioning and positions in terms of exerting a degree of control, which could also be interpreted as delaying tactics. He maintains that he will go provided 'they fit me up with a similar set of conditions to what I've got [at the current centre], practical and physical facilities, that has to be, otherwise I won't go'. This stance illustrates the point made in Chapter 5 about power. KB exerts power and he is strategically using it in a situation where the degree of power exerted by the different parties is far from equal.

Z, also from the 'innovative' residential centre, is a white man in his early twenties. He is a wheelchair user as a result of cerebral palsy. Z maintains, 'there is no option, you have to move out'. Like KB, Z has lived at the centre for a considerable time and would prefer to stay. In the text, he takes comfort from the fact that a date for moving out has not been set. He says 'no particular time's been given at the moment but you cannot stay here forever'. Moving out into the community is regarded as 'kind of scary, a bit scary'. In the text, Z can be seen to resist the position ascribed and to covertly and indirectly re-position, to prolong his stay at the centre. Accordingly he emphasises that he cannot take pressure and responds badly to it, sometimes abusing alcohol. He also talks about a 'breakdown' which he experienced, when a previous situation became too much for him to cope with. At one point in the text, he also draws attention to the fact that he cannot be offered a tenancy until he has paid off former rent arrears – something he is finding great difficulty in doing. Again Z can be seen to be responding to a situation which he finds troublesome by exerting a degree of power in a social relational context. His 'strategy' is not as consistently developed as that of Z; it is less deliberate and more emotional in tone, but he is utilising all the resources at his disposal to resist. A reading could be that emphasis on his emotional fragility, together with his highly vocal need for ongoing physical assistance, is the means to his continued residence at the centre. However, it has to be borne in mind that although Z is exerting power and drawing from available power/knowledge frameworks, he has to reduce his sights to small goals; his larger goal – to have the security of being a permanent resident in the centre – is denied him.

The ways in which privileged power/knowledge frameworks operate to legitimate a particular perspective, rendering one interpretation or view dominant and marginalising alternatives, can result in difficulties, contradictions and oppositions being ignored. There are also issues related to the information/concerns that are accepted and the information/concerns that are not (Fawcett 1998). These conceptualisations can be applied to readings of the texts. In relation to the 'traditional' residential centre, it is physical rather than psychological factors that appear to have been disproportionately attended to or 'privileged'. Accordingly, physical dependency is highlighted as the key factor in terms of who should move out and who should stay. The operation of unacknowledged dominant (and therefore privileged) power/knowledge frameworks can also be read as leading staff to ignore the ways in which the possibility of a move into the community can have a variety of meanings and implications for individuals at particular points in time. In the texts discussed above, all the residents considered their respective centres as home and all were significantly and profoundly affected by the prospect of change in a variety of different ways. In the text of Z, from the 'innovative' residential centre, for example, the prospect of a move reminds him of previous instances when pressure has been placed on him to do something that he did not want to do. Accordingly, it generates fear about living in the community related to isolation, the possibility of encountering hostile attitudes and having to cope with being 'different'. Insecurity about his future also triggers other insecurities, such as those related to his sexuality. His ambivalence about how he perceives disability and how he sees himself also come to the fore.

There are points of comparison between the ways in which Z is constructed or positioned in the text and also constructs or positions himself, and those of F from the 'traditional' residential centre. Z has actively fought changes introduced at his centre, whereas F (a 60-year-old white woman who has had rheumatoid arthritis since the age of 21) adopts a position of passive acceptance. She does not construct herself as a victim, nor as a person who has struggled against the odds, but as a person who has passively and perhaps fatalistically accepted whatever has come her way. F's passive stance towards her environment wavers, however, when she is shocked into disagreement by the prospect of change and perhaps having to move out into the community. She moves from being positioned to positioning. F is very clear that she wants to remain where she is. She does not expect that what she wants will carry any weight and her uncharacteristic verbal challenge is largely ignored. However, F's understanding of the situation is that those regarded as being most disabled and dependent will not be required to leave. Accordingly she immediately emphasises the extent of her impairment and incapacity. As far as F is concerned, 'not walking' and 'being in a chair' means that she can remain at the centre. Her impairment in this context becomes her salvation. In the text, once F positions herself in this way, her emotional intensity gives way once again to passivity and being positioned, and she reiterates a phrase she has used earlier: 'We can't say no, can we?'.

PK, also from the 'traditional' residential centre, positions himself differently. PK is a 51-year-old white man who had a stroke in 1984. The centre is his life and moving out is something he refuses to contemplate. Unlike F, he can walk and he operates as an 'honorary' member of staff. However, rather than perceiving himself to be at risk of having to move out, PK simply refuses to consider this as an option. This does not involve arguments with the centre staff, nor with representatives from the social services department; he straightforwardly ignores a move into the community as a possible option. In this, PK can be seen to occupy a strong position. Having taken on board the need to consult as promoted by the Social Services Inspectorate and other bodies (e.g. SSI/NHSME 1994, 1995; SSI 1995; SSI/Audit Commission 1996; Department of Health 1998a), representatives from the social services department would have difficulty moving an individual if that individual totally refused to either acknowledge the need for change, or to participate in the overall process. PK's position could not be seen to constitute a clear plan of action; it is clear that he just could not contemplate living anywhere else. However, of the four examples given, the positioning of PK can be viewed as the most effective. He uses day-to-day interactions and practices to resist alternative positionings.

In addition to critically interrogating privileged and dominant power/knowledge frameworks, orientations drawn from postmodern feminism(s) deconstruct the modernist view of professionals as authority figures, who, by means of their training and status, are qualified to make decisions on behalf of others. An example here relates to community care policies. In recent years, 'care management' and an emphasis on needs-led services have been regarded as key elements of community care policies facilitating service user participation. Although there are a number of approaches to and models of care management, as Payne (1995) maintains, it has been an administrative care management model based on a pro forma assessment process that has been most widely used by social services departments. As part of this process, although service users are asked to state their needs, as highlighted in Chapter 4, such 'self-assessed needs' can be seen to be managed by the assessment process, so that agency/professionally assessed needs are prioritised and legitimated.[3] As discussed above, aspects which do not fit the agency/professional assessment can easily be disregarded (Fawcett and Featherstone 1994b; Fawcett 1998). Orientations derived from postmodern feminism(s) emphasise that all power/knowledge claims can be weighted in particular contexts and that although certain perspectives aspire to dominance, there can be no foundationalist basis for such claims. In turn, the viewing of service user perspectives as 'innocent' and the privileging of these perspectives as a means of countering professional dominance is also critiqued. Emphasis is therefore placed on negotiation in specific contexts, with all parties being viewed as important participators in the process. Accordingly, categorisation procedures which, for example, fail to fully acknowledge disabled women and men as multifaceted individuals, have also to be recognised and addressed. The posing, either directly or indirectly, of binary oppositions between, for example, disabled service users and agency/professionals are similarly rejected.

Chapter 4 highlighted the tensions between the implementation of top-down management performance systems within social services departments and the greater involvement of service users in planning forums and in determining how self-assessed needs can be met. Orientations drawn from postmodern feminism(s) suggest that tensions, clearly specified, can be productive. In any interaction, in any context, there will be differing agendas operating. The exploration and acknowledgement of such tensions by all involved parties can result in courses of action which facilitate all parties getting something of what they want, whilst at the same time contributing to related debates in different arenas. An example that takes account of the current community care climate in Britain could relate to a woman recently impaired by means of a leg amputation, having her self-defined need for person-centred counselling met from a budget monitored by a performance indicator focusing on the amount of physical assistance provided by home-care workers in a given period. In turn, the social services department could use this flexibility as evidence of how it actively involves service users in tailoring individual packages of care. Both could then present the case for a locally agreed performance indicator focusing on the meeting of counselling needs.

Perspectives emanating from postmodern feminism(s) also highlight contradictions and areas of omission. These areas are often not attended to in accounts which seek to provide a rational explanation or to present a rounded picture. People do not behave in clear and rational ways, although often disabled women and men feel that they have to account for themselves in accordance with such linearly framed criteria. An example could be interaction between a disabled woman and a care manager. The woman may not feel that it 'fits' her account to talk about how her impairment causes her abilities to fluctuate during the day. She may feel that she will be responded to unfavourably if she explains that although she can usually make breakfast for herself in the morning and sometimes at lunch-time, there are periods when she feels unable to deal with a kettle full of boiling water. She may also feel it unacceptable, if a trip to the shops with a voluntary worker is arranged, to specify how she has to plan any trip out around the availability of accessible toilets. Attention to complexity, contradiction and paradox can be seen to be features that promote an inclusive rather than an exclusive approach to disability, and this is an area that will be returned to in the concluding section of this chapter.

Multiple selves

Orientations derived from postmodern feminism(s) highlight that the subject positions adopted, and also the ways in which subjects are positioned, are often multiple and contradictory. A disabled woman, for example, may be a strong adherent of the social model of disability, yet there will be times when she uses her impairment to obtain a response or treatment that could be regarded as different and favourable. There will be other times when she campaigns strongly for accessible and height-sensitive working environments, others when she operates as a mother, others as a respected academic and so on. As discussed in Chapter 5, an individual can be seen to have a shifting 'core' which continually changes, making it possible to relate to different people in different situations in different ways. The 'self' in accordance with perspectives emanating from postmodern feminism(s) is a social self, and interaction necessitates the adoption of a wide range of responses and personas. In some, disability might feature strongly, in others feminist perspectives, in yet others those of a daughter, or grandmother, or confidante. All engaged in social interaction always have alternative positions to occupy and explore.

A central application of perspectives derived from postmodern feminism(s) discussed throughout this book is the emphasis placed on a subject being both constructed and capable of construction and critique. It is useful at this point to illustrate this aspect more fully, by reference to the research study mentioned earlier (Fawcett 1999b) in relation to how a subject could be positioned with regard to 'medical models' of disability and also the social model.

MP lives in the community. She is a 58-year-old white woman who lives alone. She became a wheelchair user in 1983 as a result of rheumatoid arthritis and spinal problems. MP constructs herself as a clear thinking, intelligent, aware person, who wants to obtain a reasonable quality of life both for herself and for other disabled people. She is keen not to criticise individuals, but cites planners, and by implication bureaucracies, as not being aware of the real difficulties that disabled people face. She highlights that what appears to be a small and rather insignificant problem to an able-bodied person can appear to be a huge difficulty to a disabled person to the extent that their mental health is affected. An example she gives relates to cleaning. 'Care' services no longer provide cleaning and MP says that she finds having to contemplate dirty windows or a dirty carpet all day frustrating and demoralising. She also refers to how in the winter she has to spend all day looking at the muddy footprints left by the 'care' worker. With regard to 'medical models', MP could be constructed as being awkward, demanding and as not considering others in similar if not worse situations sufficiently. She could also be positioned as a woman who is astutely pointing to deficiencies in a system that is starved of resources. In relation to the social model of disability, she could be constructed as an informed woman who knows best how her needs could be met and who is striving to achieve as much autonomy and control as her 'care' situation will allow.

BP, also from the community, is a 21-year-old black man who has lived in Britain for 18 months. He has been a wheelchair user for the past eight years and makes it clear that he does not position himself as a disabled person. According to BP, disabled people are people who cannot 'do' things for themselves, but he makes it clear by reference to his 'independence', ability to think, academic qualifications and sporting abilities that he '*can* do' and is different. The emphasis presented is of an active, doing individual, yet there are times in the next when the 'I can' construction is subject to qualification. For example, rather than talking about a need for 'care' or personal assistance, BP reframes his needs in terms of only wanting help for things he cannot do himself. It becomes clear that there are a large number of things that BP requires assistance with (e.g. washing, showering, washing clothes, making meals) but his construction of himself emphasises what he can do. In accordance with 'medical model' scenarios, BP could be positioned as a 'heroic survivor'. In turn, the social model of disability could position him as an individual who denies impairment, does not challenge disablism but seeks identification with 'normal people' and who seeks to reinforce this role through his sporting activities.

Risks, expertise and ethics

In Chapter 2, notions of risk were appraised. In the light of a discussion highlighting applications drawn from postmodern feminism(s), it is possible to question current notions of risk and risk assessment and to view these as being underpinned by concepts of objectivity and rationality. Views of risk, as discussed in Chapter 2, are subject to prevailing values and prioritisations and can be positioned both culturally and historically. This is not to dismiss risk assessment *per se*, but to acknowledge that there are no certainties and that context and the weighted interactions of those present have to play a key role. In relation to discussions about disability and challenging behaviour, for example, the drawing up of pro forma procedural documents for workers to assiduously follow, has to be viewed extremely cautiously. Competency based training is currently in vogue for those working in social and health care, yet drawing from orientations emanating from postmodern feminism(s), it can be seen to be important for workers to be able to weigh up particular situations, using knowledge that is context-specific and that which is transferable between contexts. It is also helpful to engage positively, to interact effectively and to avoid establishing professional/worker versus individual with challenging behaviour binaries. Placing workers in the position of technicians following instructions can be viewed as unhelpful, possibly even dangerous. Of course it is possible to argue at this point (as many working in this arena would) that procedures are for guidance only and that professional expertise is used to make specific decisions and to decide upon particular courses of action. However, Jan Fook (1999) draws attention to how professional practice and expertise have been challenged by technocratisation and the devaluing of professional knowledge and skills. The operation in social and health care services of the purchaser–provider split has meant that the power for policy-making is removed from professionals with specific expertise. Instead there is a managerial culture within which control is maintained through procedural practice guidance and competitive and short-term contractual funding arrangements. In such a climate, recourse to 'professional expertise' can be seen to be time-limited.

In addition, as discussed previously, the whole notion of 'professional expertise' is questioned by postmodern perspectives. However, drawing from postmodern feminism(s), Fook (1999) makes suggestions which not only reconceptualise notions of expertise, but also serve as a point of challenge to postmodernist divisions in the field of knowledge reproduction. Such reformulations include an emphasis on contextuality, which refers to the ability to work in and with the whole context or situation, appreciating fully the influence of differing and competing factors. Contextuality, in turn, involves a form of connectedness in that connections are made with the viewpoints and experiences of others. Knowledge and theory creation are also viewed as interactive and ongoing. Accordingly, emphasis is placed on transferable rather than generalisable knowledge and upon creating new knowledge that is not only situation-specific but which also feeds into transferable knowledge. Matters of process also become key, as workers negotiate and interact with all those involved. The importance of critical reflexivity is additionally highlighted, as workers review, challenge and reformulate their knowledge/power understandings in a grounded context. Fook (1999) maintains that such a reformulation facilitates the creation of critical knowledge that potentially challenges and resists current forms of domination whilst maintaining commitment to a system of social values that allows social and health care staff to work with, yet transcend, the contradictions and uncertainties of daily practice (Fook 1999).

The implication for disabled people is that it becomes possible to breach the divides between professionals and disabled service users. If we are all viewed as having impairments, but with some impairments related to our bodies and our minds being more obvious or serious or enduring than others, then professionality has to be reconceptualised so that negotiation, interaction, contextuality, transferability, reflexivity and process become key attributes.

In relation to reformulations drawn from postmodern feminism(s), it is also important to consider questions of ethics. Ethics, defined as criteria which guide how we act, have occupied a central position in feminism(s), and feminist exposures of discriminatory and oppressive practices have been clearly seen as part of a feminist ethical code. However, notions of ethics can be seen to be firmly located within modernist frameworks and ideas of moral development. As Rossiter *et al.* (1999) highlight, many considerations of ethics (e.g. Trevino) rest on views of the liberal humanist individual who possesses particular internal characteristics and who, as a result of high levels of ego strength, field independence and a strong internal locus of control, is deemed to be in a position to operate ethically. Rossiter *et al.* (1999) point to how conceptualisations of such an individual equate with autonomous, independent, masculine ideals of the Enlightenment. Modernist feminism(s), although incorporating deconstructive and focused critiques, can also be seen to rely on liberal humanist and individually orientated underpinnings. Orientations emanating from postmodern feminism(s), although retaining the critically deconstructive edge of modernist feminism(s), can be seen to have moved on from an understanding of ethics as the property of individuals to view ethics as social relations that affect ethical decision-making. As Rossiter *et al.* (1999) maintain, an implication of this shift is that ongoing attention has to be paid to communicative processes. It has also to be acknowledged that a consideration of ethics relates to a much broader set of activities than is associated with conventional understandings. They assert that the question 'who is afraid to speak and why?' is a means of keeping ethics at the centre of professional and social practices. They draw attention to matters of process and contend that local, particular, historical and contingent dilemmas require an ongoing process of critique from the perspective of the present. As previously highlighted, the paying of continual attention to how process issues may exclude certain individuals, has a particular relevance for interaction in the field of disability.

The weighting of oppressions

It is also useful to elaborate further at this point on the practical applicability of perspectives drawn from postmodern feminism(s) to issues of oppression. Hearn and Parkin (1993), focusing on organisations, multiple oppressions and postmodernism, maintain that an exploration of the construction of disability and ability highlights underlying issues relating to the organisational construction of the perception of the senses in terms of who possesses these and how they are valued. This is turn can be associated with constructions of knowledge. In the texts generated by the research study alluded to earlier (Fawcett 1999), the knowledge base of the subjects can be seen to be devalued on the basis of an able-bodied, hierarchically organised knowledge framework.

In a consideration of oppressions, it is important to re-emphasise that orientations emanating from postmodern feminism(s) do not dismiss the recognition of oppressions as part of modernist projects, nor reduce oppression to a consideration of difference, but focus on how oppressions can be seen to be interrelated and continually produced and reproduced by means of discursive practices (Hearn and Parkin 1993). Although particular contexts are seen as important, the making of inter-contextual connections is viewed as equally significant and as a means of not relegating issues of oppression to relativistic obscurity. A matter referred to earlier in this chapter can be used as an example. With regard to the research project (Fawcett 1999b), the texts of subjects from the 'innovative' residential centre and the 'traditional' residential centre focused on having to move out of their respective centres. Here, the possible loss of what the subjects regard as 'their home' featured significantly. It is also a point of note that the respondents from the 'innovative' residential centre, despite a greater familiarity with the social model of disability, found themselves in the same position as their counterparts from the 'traditional' residential centre in relation to a lack of control over the making of key decisions. The ways in which the texts in relation to this issue may be seen to interconnect, can in turn be linked to the manner in which the various social services departments dismissed these concerns and pressed on with their policies. The textual interconnections facilitate the identification of an oppressive practice that can be associated with further oppressions related to disablism and the hegemony of able-bodied knowledge claims. The identification of this practice, seen from the texts to be generalised rather than specific, facilitates the deconstruction of the underpinning knowledge frameworks.

Bodily considerations

Applications emanating from postmodern feminism(s) reject mind/body dualisms and draw attention to the variety of ways in which bodies are viewed, responded to and used. As discussed in Chapters 2 and 5, bodies, particularly impaired bodies, are frequently subject to negative positionings. Writers such as Oliver (1996) and Shakespeare (1996) have emphasised that a medicalised focus on impairment (viewed as disability) almost inevitably leads to a negative self-image. However, orientations drawn from postmodern feminism draw attention to how constructions of 'self' fluctuate in different contexts. The research project referred to earlier (Fawcett 1999b), for example, found that just under half of the respondents in the context of the interview projected a positive self-image that fully incorporated impairment. Only 2 out of 25 respondents who saw impairment as an indivisible part of their sense of 'self' projected negative self-images. Both of these respondents were experi-encing rapid deterioration with regard to their impairments and it was this, rather than other factors, that influenced how they currently saw themselves. Accordingly, with regard to postmodern feminism, straightforward associations are rejected in favour of a 'both and' form of analysis which takes contextual variations fully into account.

Concluding remarks

In this chapter the possible utility of orientations derived from postmodern feminism(s) has been considered. It is possible to assert that such applications contribute towards an inclusive rather than an exclusive view of disability. Accordingly, modernist under-standings of needs, rights and citizenship can be reformulated and related to specific contexts, difference can be viewed as a resource and the temporary fixing of difference to make political challenges can be highlighted. Privileged knowledge frameworks can be decon-structed and the ways in which varying perspectives can operate in differing contexts can be explored. Additionally, there is a focus on 'multiple selves', and subjectivity, as comprising a shifting 'core' which is fully cognisant of social interrelationships. Notions of risk and professional/agency expertise and ethics can be reappraised and problems associated with rational underpinnings can be highlighted. Oppressions can be seen as being interrelated and as being continually reproduced and open to challenge in different contexts. With regard to bodies, binary pairing can be rejected in favour of inclusive 'both and' forms of analysis.

Summary

- The applicability of orientations emanating from postmodern feminism(s) has been explored in relation to debates and discussions in the field of disability.

- Ways in which postmodern perspectives challenge modernist conceptions of needs, rights and citizenship have been emphasised and the part which postmodern feminism(s) can play in utilisable reformulations has been explored.

- The ways in which perspectives derived from postmodern feminism(s) place emphasis on the identification of privileged power/knowledge frameworks, and on the manner in which these operate, have been highlighted. Subjects can be seen to be positioned in particular ways by the operation of power/knowledge frameworks, or subjects can position, utilising the power/knowledge frameworks available, in indirect, direct, covert or overt ways.

- Drawing from postmodern feminism, notions of the 'self' have been seen to be multiple and contradictory. A person can be seen to have a shifting 'core' that continually changes, making it possible to relate to different people in different situations in different ways, depending upon context.

- In a discussion of risks, expertise and ethics, perspectives emanating from postmodern feminism(s) have been used to question an emphasis on rationality and to promote orientations that focus on context, process and critical reflexivity.

- With regard to a consideration of oppressions, orientations emanating from postmodern feminism(s) have been used to make connections. Accordingly, the recognition of oppressions is not dismissed as part of a modernist project, nor is it reduced to a consideration of difference. Instead there is an emphasis on how oppressions can be seen to be interrelated and continually produced and reproduced by means of discursive practices. Although particular contexts are important, the making of inter-contextual connections is viewed as equally significant and as a means of not relegating issues of oppression to relativistic obscurity.

- Applications emanating from postmodern feminism(s) have also been seen to reject mind/body dualisms and to draw attention to the many diverse ways in which bodies can be viewed, responded to and used.

Notes

1 The term 'reformulation(s)' is used here to refer to perspectives drawn from postmodern feminism(s). It is employed as a shorthand term and is not meant to imply the presentation of a 'grandnarrative', nor that the orientations emanating from postmodern feminism(s) can be seen as unitary and consistent.

2 For Flax (1992b), reconciliation refers to an ongoing 'unity of differences' which feature mutuality and incorporation rather than the annihilation of opposites and distinctions. Reciprocity relates to an emphasis on the sharing of authority and a mutuality in decision-making processes in the absence of dominating perspectives of 'objective standards' or 'normative practices' (Flax 1992b: 206). Recognition is about accepting and positively regarding differentness whilst simultaneously recognising sameness in terms of how the other is like oneself. Judgement, in turn, highlights connectedness and obligation to others and the quality of care that arises out of this.

3 With regard to agency/professionally assessed need, the debates about the extent to which 'new managerialism' (e.g. Clarke 1996) and community care policies have stripped social workers of claims to 'professionalism', substituting instead agency-dominated agendas, are accepted.

Further reading

Fawcett, B., Featherstone, B., Fook, J. and Rossiter, A. (eds) (1999) *Researching and Practising in Social Work: Postmodern Feminist Perspectives*, London: Routledge.

Flax, J. (1992) 'Beyond Equality, Gender, Justice and Difference' in Bock, L. and James, S. (eds) *Beyond Equality and Difference*, London: Routledge, pp. 193–210.

Hearn, J. (1998) 'Theorising Men and Men's Theorising: Varieties of Discursive Practices in Men's Theorising of Men' in *Theory and Society*, **27**(6): 781–816.

Nicholson, L. and Seidman, S. (eds) (1995) *Social Postmodernism: Beyond Identity Politics*, Cambridge: Cambridge University Press.

Chapter 7

Conclusion

Chapter outline

This short concluding chapter reviews the following:

- the arguments presented with regard to how perspectives drawn from postmodern feminism(s) can be used to explore tensions and make links between modernism and postmodernism
- similarities and differences between postmodern feminism(s) and other perspectives which seek to make connections between agency and structure
- the contribution that postmodern feminism(s) can make to debates in the field of disability

Introduction

In this book it has been argued that feminist perspectives can be used as a point of comparison and also as a critical tool to appraise developments in the field of disability such as the social model. This is not to devalue the social model. On the contrary, the ways in which this model, with its clear political agenda, has radically changed thinking around disability and has led to significant developments in terms of policy and practice, has to be fully acknowledged. The comparisons from feminism(s) have been used to highlight similarities in both emancipatory movements and to identify possible problem areas for the further development of the social model and associated disability rights campaigns.

Orientations emanating from postmodern feminism(s) have been explored in order to offer further theoretical and practical insights and applications that could have a bearing on developments in the field of disability. The intention is not to use these perspectives to contest the social model, nor to set up an alternative framework, but to add to the debates and discussions currently taking place.

As seen in Chapter 5, postmodern feminism(s) can be used to critically appraise aspects of modernism and postmodernism and to explore tensions and make links between the perspectives. To summarise briefly, in relation to modernism, postmodern feminism(s) highlights the tensions associated with an emphasis on progress and on the importance attached to rational and objective underpinnings for ideas and actions. Tensions related to structural frameworks, which are inextricably interrelated with big stories or metanarratives (such as humanism, liberalism, feminism(s) and the social model of disability) and which use structuralist, materialist arguments to press for change, are similarly emphasised. Universally applicable theoretical perspectives, such as psychoanalysis, and an emphasis on economic determinism are additionally regarded as problematic. Similarly, modernity's faith in science, the possibility of discovering the truth of any situation and an emphasis on binary pairings such as nature/culture, superstition/rationality, body/mind, able-bodiedness/disabled-bodiedness, are rejected. There is also a focus on the tensions associated with modernist views of an essentialist, unified, coherent 'core' self, where individual thinking informs action and where language reflects individually created meanings and something 'real'.

With regard to postmodernism, postmodern feminism(s) emphasises the tensions contained within the promotion of anti-foundationalist thinking, which makes it difficult, if not impossible, to ground any ideas or to make distinctions between what is acceptable and what is not. The relativity embedded in such anti-foundationalist thinking renders the identification of inequalities and the mounting of effective challenges extremely difficult. If all ideas and actions are relative, then none can carry more weight than any other and issues relating to disablism and sexism can be dismissed as irrelevant. Tensions contained within a postmodernism emphasis on superficiality over depth are also foregrounded by postmodern feminism(s). Within postmodernism, glossy magazines, for example, are viewed as being as important as literary works and a focus on pluralism and pragmatism ensures that 'anything goes'. Tensions embedded in views of the 'self' as fluid, as a creation of language or discourse and as a socially constructed entity that lacks agency, are also acknowledged.

This overview is somewhat brief and in emphasising the tensions associated with modern and postmodern perspectives, negative rather than positive aspects of both have been highlighted. However, perspectives that draw from postmodern feminism(s) recognise useful as well as problematic areas. Postmodern feminism(s) therefore draws from both to make links which, it is argued, have a theoretical and practical relevance for debates relating to the field of disability.

As discussed in Chapter 5 in relation to knowledge and power, both modernist foundational and postmodernist anti-foundationalist conceptualisations are rejected, but links are made in the ways that all power/knowledge claims are viewed as privileged and non-innocent. However, the possibility of weighting conflicting claims in particular contexts is retained. The making of inter-contextual connections also becomes possible in that the manner in which oppressions, manifested in particular contexts, are continually produced and reproduced by means of discursive practices can be highlighted. With regard to subjectivity and views of the self, links are made by not privileging experience and regarding it as unique, nor promoting understandings of the 'self' as the same irrespective of context. Instead, emphasis is placed on the 'self' as a fluid, social entity who is constructed and positioned by social practices and discursive interplay, but who can also position and critique. With regard to matters of difference, modernist emphases on fixed differences, which can so easily slide into divisions with attendant inequalities, and postmodernist concerns with pluralism and relativity, are reformulated. Accordingly, it is seen to be possible to temporarily freeze differences in order to explore commonalities and to engage in political action (F. Williams 1996). Such temporary freezing of difference facilitates movement between different groupings and coalitions, depending upon the various agendas operating, and militates against rigidity and the development of foundationalist underpinnings. In relation to conceptualisations of able-bodiedness, disabled-bodiedness and the body, modernist mind/body, able-bodied/disabled-bodied binaries are eschewed and links are made by emphasising 'both and' rather than 'either or' formulations. Accordingly, if a disabled person wants to fully embrace the social model of disability, yet at times still play a role that would be viewed by proponents of the social model of disability as that of 'heroic victim', then according to reformulations drawing from postmodern feminism(s), both positionings would be possible. Notions of the body are also not subject to mind/body binary separations and bodies are seen as both being inscribed and capable of inscription.

The overview given above shows how perspectives derived from postmodern feminism(s) can be used, and their applicability to the field of disability has been reviewed in Chapter 6. However, a key feature of the arguments presented has related to issues of individual intentionality or agency, and discursive positioning. With regard to the theoretical discussions contained in Chapter 5, subjects have been regarded as being constructed and positioned, and capable of construction, positioning and critique. There are echoes here of debates contained within a modernist frame relating to agency and structure and it is useful, at this concluding stage, to briefly explore similarities and differences between the arguments presented in this book and formulations such as that of structuration theory expounded by Giddens (1984, 1991). The areas considered will relate to power/knowledge frameworks and the ways in which social practices are influenced, notions of subjectivity and the 'self', and features relating to individual agency (or intentionally) and structural (and discursive) influences.

Postmodern feminism(s) and structuration theory

Giddens (1984), by means of structuration theory and the notion of a duality of structure, postulates a view that emphasises the interrelationship between social structure and individual action. Social practices are seen as integral to the duality of structure in that it is in social practices that the interplay of action and structure occurs. Action and structure are regarded as forming different aspects of social practices (Bauman 1992; Layder 1994). Giddens' view of social practices does not accord with that of Foucault (1979, 1981a,b, 1986) in that Giddens does not view social practices as constructs, rather as manifestations of the actions of unique individual agents who intentionally and unintentionally both modify and reproduce acquired practices and knowledge frameworks. However, there are some points of overlap with orientations drawn from postmodern feminism(s) which emphasise that subjects are both constructed and capable of construction and critique, in that Giddens (1991) refers to self-identity as being reflexive in terms of

the 'self' not being viewed as static, but revised in relation to changing circumstances. However, a major point of difference relates to
the emphasis that Giddens (1984) places on the 'unique' actions
of individual agents and on their possession of a coherent identity,
where an individual's sense of self follows their changing bio-
graphical narrative (Giddens 1984, 1991; Layder 1994). These differences become more pronounced in that with regard to notions
of subjectivity and the 'self', Giddens regards human agents as
possessing different levels of consciousness. These levels include
an unconscious motivational level, a practical level, which refers to
knowing how to act in a range of social situations, and a structural
or discursive consciousness. In relation to the latter, however, there
are again some points of overlap with orientations drawn from
postmodern feminism(s) in that Giddens (1984, 1991) maintains
that although individual agents use and exert power, their agency
can be limited by the entrenchment of various forms of domination
which, together with the view that people do not create society
but reproduce what is already there, places limitations on possible
actions and on individual agency. Additional similarities can also
be discerned in that Giddens' (1984) conceptualisation of power
appears to be relational, rather than absolute, with individuals, by
means of 'the dialectics of control', having at their disposal a variety
of resources, with the balance of power relating to access to resources of power in particular contexts. By his references to 'locale',
i.e. the points where physical space intersects with social practices,
he also highlights the importance of context.

However, although, arguably, there can be seen to be some
points of overlap between structuration theory and orientations
emanating from postmodern feminism(s) in that structuration
theory highlights the importance of 'locale' or context, focuses on
dynamic selves who change according to context and discusses the
perpetration of social practices which limit agency, it is the differences that predominate. These relate to the disproportionate
emphasis placed on individual agency, a coherent identity and
aspects of social reality which can be looked at objectively by human
agents. Gendered perspectives do not tend to feature significantly
in structuration theory, and the ways in which the unequal distribu-
tion of resources reflect and reinforce the general power structure
and entrenched social divisions can also be seen to be insufficiently
addressed (Layder 1994; Scott 1995).

The above discussion can be seen as a useful way of highlighting the ways in which the perspectives drawn from postmodern

feminism(s) and utilised in this book both relate to and also differ from theoretical perspectives which arguably have explored some similar key areas.

Concluding remarks

Consider the following extracts from Shakespeare's *The Tempest*:

Miranda about Ferdinand:

> I might call him
> A thing divine; for nothing natural
> I ever saw so noble.

Prospero about Caliban:

> A devil, a born devil, on whose nature
> Nurture can never stick; on whom my pains,
> Humanely taken, all, all lost, quite lost:
> And as, with age, his body uglier grows,
> So his mind cankers.

The above quotes refer to a description of a 'normal' human male by the lovelorn Miranda and a description of a deformed being, a 'monster' by Prospero, Miranda's father. Arguably, for those familiar with the play, Prospero was provoked into such a vehement rejection of Caliban, by Caliban's attempted rape of his daughter. However, Caliban's bodily form is seen to reflect his inner imperfect state and these quotes can be seen as examples of normatively, negatively framed difference, which still have resonance today. The social model of disability has very successfully challenged normatively and negatively framed differences between able-bodied and disabled-bodied women and men and the ways in which this is manifested in individual, social and institutional practices. However, within disability rights campaigns based on the social model of disability, there can be seen to be problem areas related to the machinations of identity politics, experiential validation and marginalisation. The social model of disability has also run into difficulties when it comes to acknowledging and creatively and non-divisively responding to differences amongst disabled people.

It has been contended in this book that orientations emanating from postmodern feminism can be used as critical and creative tools and that these perspectives have something useful to offer to debates in the field of disability. However, with regard to both theoretical discussions and applications, it has to be stated that the intention is not to devalue the contribution of the social model of disability, nor to undermine its importance and achievements. The purpose of applying perspectives drawn from postmodern feminism(s) has been to explore tensions and make links between modernism and postmodernism and in so doing to respond to postmodern critiques of modern, structuralist positions, such as the social model of disability, and to contribute towards ongoing debates and discussions.

With regard to the disability arena, it has to be emphasised that perspectives derived from postmodern feminism(s) cannot be used to produce an alternative definition of disability, one that attempts to address the gaps and silences in the social model and rectify deficiencies in 'medical models'. The orientations utilised cannot give an exact meaning or a precise definition of disability, nor provide a summary of the particular components or properties involved. However, the analysis presented can be employed to give an interpretation of disability where the impossibility of producing a precise definition can be seen to be productive, challenging and creative. In such an inclusive interpretation, exclusive, fixed positions, rigid certainties and privileged linearly framed explanations, prescriptions and solutions are eschewed. Instead, there is a focus on factors relating to identity, experience, categorisation processes and group membership being always in process. This is not to argue for ongoing relativity and a total fluidity of positions. Rather the aim, with regard to the analysis presented and the links made, is to relate definitions, meanings, actions and challenges to specific situations where ongoing negotiation, facilitation and pragmatic groupings or coalitions become the defining features. Accordingly, positions can be temporarily adopted and plans made and carried through, but on the understanding that there are other positions, other plans and that the definitions and action strategies adopted at a particular point in time are always open to change.

Summary

- Ways of exploring tensions and making links between modern and postmodern perspectives utilising orientations drawn from postmodern feminism have been reviewed.

- Points of overlap between structuration theory, as devised by Giddens (1984, 1991), and postmodern feminism have been explored. Some points of overlap relating to the importance both perspectives ascribe to 'locale' or context, the emphasis placed on dynamic selves who change according to context, and the perpetration of social practices which limit agency, can be discerned, but it is the differences associated with the disproportionate emphasis placed on individual agency, a coherent identity and aspects of social reality that can be looked at objectively by human agents in structuration theory, which predominate.

The strengths and problem areas associated with the social model of disability have been highlighted and the contribution which postmodern feminism(s) can make has been appraised. In this context, the analysis presented, which draws from postmodern feminism, can be used to present an interpretation of disability where the impossibility of producing a precise definition can be seen as productive. Such an inclusive interpretation places emphasis on process, negotiation and pragmatic coalitions or groupings working at particular points in time towards specific goals.

Further reading

Giddens, A. (1984) *The Constitution of Society*, Cambridge: Polity Press.

Giddens, A. (1991) *Modernity and Self Identity*, Cambridge: Polity Press.

Bibliography

Abberley, P. (1987) 'The Concept of Oppression and the Development of a Social Theory of Disability' in *Disability, Handicap and Society*, **2**(1): 5–21.

Abberley, P. (1997) 'The Limits of Classical Social Theory in the Analysis and Transformation of Disablement (Can This Really Be the End; To Be Stuck Inside of Mobile With The Memphis Blues Again?)' in Barton, L. and Oliver, M. (eds) *Disability Studies: Past, Present and Future*, Leeds: The Disability Press, pp. 25–44.

Abrams, P., Abrams, S., Humphrey, R. and Smith, R. (1989) *Neighbourhood Care and Social Policy*, London: HMSO.

Abu-Habib, L. (1997) *Gender and Disability: Women's Experiences in the Middle East*, Oxford: Oxfam Publications.

Adams, M. L. (1989) 'There's No Place Like Home: On the Place of Identity in Feminist Politics' in *Feminist Review*, **31** (Spring): 23–33.

Alcoff, L. (1988) 'Poststructuralism and Cultural Feminism' in *Signs*, **13**: 5–36.

Alibhai, Y. (1999) *Beyond Black and White*, Radio 4, 5 March 1999.

Almond, B. (1993) 'Rights' in Singer, P. (ed.) *A Companion to Ethics*, Oxford: Blackwell, pp. 259–69.

Althusser, L. (1971) *Lenin and Philosophy and Other Essays*, London: New Left Books.

Arber, S. and Gilbert, N. (1993) 'Men: The Forgotten Carers' in Bornat, J., Pereira, C., Pilgrim, D. and Williams, F. (eds) *Community Care: A Reader*, Basingstoke: Open University/Macmillan, pp. 134–42.

Arber, S. and Ginn, J. (1990) 'The Meaning of Informal: Gender and the Contribution of Elderly People', *Ageing and Society*, **10**(4): 429–54.

Arber, S. and Ginn, J. (eds) (1995) *Connecting Gender and Ageing: A Sociological Approach*, Buckingham: Open University Press.

Ardill, S. and O'Sullivan, S. (1986) 'Upsetting an Applecart: Difference, Desire and Lesbian Sadomasochism' in *Feminist Review*, **23** (June): 31–56.

Arney, W. R. and Bergen, B. J. (1983) 'The Anomaly of the Chronic Patient and the Play of Medical Power' in *Sociology of Health and Illness*, **5**(1): 1–24.

Atkar, S., Ghataora, R. with Baldwin, N. and Thanki, V. (1997) *Hifazat-Surukhia: Keeping Safe*, Halesowen: NSPCC/University of Warwick/University of Dundee.

Baistow, K. (1994) 'Liberation and Regulation: Some Paradoxes of Empowerment' in *Critical Social Policy*, **42** (Winter 1994/1995): 34–46.

Baldock, J. and Ungerson, C. (1994) 'A Consumer View of the New Community Care: The Home Care Experiences of a Sample of Stroke Survivors and Their Carers in Care in Place' in *The International Journal of Networks and Community*, **1**(2): 175–87.

Balloch, S. (1999) 'What the Paper Says' in *Community Care Magazine*, 4–10 March 1999, p. 21.

Barnes, C. (1990) *Cabbage Syndrome: The Social Construction of Dependency*, London: Falmer Press.

Barnes, C. (1997a) 'A Legacy of Oppression: A History of Disability in Western Culture' in Barton, L. and Oliver, M. (eds) *Disability Studies: Past, Present and Future*, Leeds: The Disability Press, pp. 3–24.

Barnes, C. (1997b) 'The Social Model of Disability: A Sociological Phenomenon Ignored by Sociologists', Paper Presented at British Sociological Association Conference, April 1997.

Barnes, C. and Mercer, G. (eds) (1996) *Exploring the Divide: Illness and Disability*, Leeds: The Disability Press.

Barnes, C. and Mercer, G. (eds) (1997) *Doing Disability Research*, Leeds: The Disability Press.

Barnes, C., Mercer, G. and Shakespeare, T. (1999) *Exploring Disability: A Sociological Introduction*, Cambridge: Polity Press.

Barnes, H., Thornton, P. and Maynard Cambell, S. (1998) *Disabled People and Employment: A Review of Research and Development Work*, West Sussex: J. R. Rowntree Foundation and Policy Press.

Barnes, M. (1997) *Care, Communities and Citizens*, London: Longman.

Barrett, M. (1987) 'The Concept of Difference' in *Feminist Review*, **26**: 29–41.

Barrett, M. (1991) *The Politics of Truth: From Marx to Foucault*, Cambridge: Polity Press.

Barrett, M. (1992) 'Words and Things: Materialism and Method in Contemporary Feminist Analysis' in Barrett, M. and Phillips, A. (eds) *Destabilising Theory: Contemporary Feminist Debates*, Cambridge: Polity Press, pp. 201–19.

Barrett, M. and McIntosh, M. (1982) *The Anti-social Family*, London: Verso.

Barrett, M. and Phillips, A. (eds) (1992) *Destabilising Theory: Contemporary Feminist Debates*, Cambridge: Polity Press.

Bartky, S. L. (1988) 'Foucault, Femininity, and the Modernization of Patriarchial Power' in Diamond, I. and Quinby, L. (eds) *Feminism and Foucault*, Boston: Northeastern University Press.

Barton, L. (ed.) (1996) *Disability and Society: Emerging Issues and Insights*, London: Longman.

Barton, L. and Oliver, M. (eds) (1997) *Disability Studies: Past, Present and Future*, Leeds: The Disability Press.

Bauman, Z. (1992) *Intimations of Postmodernity*, London: Routledge.

Bayley, M. (1973) *Mental Handicap and Community Care*, London: Routledge and Kegan Paul.

Beardshaw, V. and Towell, D. (1990) *Assessment and Care Management: Implications for the Implementation of 'Caring for People'*, London: Kings Fund Institute Briefing Paper 10.

Beauvoir, Simone de (1953) *The Second Sex*, New York: Alfred A. Knopf.

Begum, N. (1992) 'Disabled Women and the Feminist Agenda' in *Feminist Review*, **40**: 70–84.

Begum, N., Hill, M. and Stevens, A. (eds) (1994) *Reflections: The Views of Black Disabled People on their Lives and Community Care*, London: Central Council for Education and Training in Social Work, Paper 32.3.

Benhabib, S. (1992) *Situating the Self. Gender, Community and Postmodernism in Contemporary Ethics*, London: Routledge.

Benhabib, S. (1995) 'Feminism and Postmodernism' in Nicholson, L. (ed.) *Feminist Contentions: A Philosophical Exchange*, London: Routledge, pp. 17–34.

Benhabib, S. and Cornell, D. (1987) *Feminism as Critique*, Cambridge: Polity Press.

Beresford, P. (1999) 'Review of Modernising Social Services White Paper' in *Community Care Magazine*, 11–17 March 1999.

Beresford, P. and Croft, S. (1993) *Citizen Involvement: A Practical Guide for Change*, Basingstoke: BASW/Macmillan.

Beresford, P. and Trevillion, S. (1995) *Developing Skills for Community Care: A Collaborative Approach*, Aldershot: Arena.

Berger, P. and Luckmann, T. (1966) *The Social Construction of Reality: A Treatise in the Sociology of Knowledge*, London: Penguin.

Best, S. and Kellner, D. (1991) *Postmodern Theory: Critical Interrogations*, Basingstoke: Macmillan.

Bhavnani, K. K. (1993) 'Tracing the Contours: Feminist Research and Feminist Objectivity' in *Women's Studies International Forum*, **16**(2): 95–104.

Blair, M. and Holland, J. with Sheldon, S. (eds) (1995) *Identity and Diversity: Gender and the Experience of Education*, Clevedon: Multilingual Matters in association with the Open University Press.

Bock, G. and James, S. (eds) (1992) *Beyond Equality and Difference*, London: Routledge.

Bokhari, S., Khan, S., Sagoo, K. and Race, T. (1996) *Report of Research Project to Evaluate the Needs of Asian Children who have been Sexually Abused in Bradford*, Bradford: Bradford Family Service Unit/Bradford Health Ethnic Minority Health Fund.

Boniface, D. and Denham, M. (1997) 'Factors Influencing the Use of Community Health and Social Services by Those Aged Sixty Five and Over' in *Health and Social Care in the Community*, 5(1): 48–54.

Bordo, S. (1993) 'Feminism, Foucault and the Politics of the Body' in Ramazanoğlu, C. (ed.) *Up Against Foucault: Explorations of Some Tensions Between Foucault and Feminism*, London: Routledge, pp. 179–202.

Borsay, A. (1997) 'Personal Trouble or Public Issue' in Barton, L. and Oliver, M. (eds) *Disability Studies: Past, Present and Future*, Leeds: The Disability Press.

Boyne, R. and Rattansi, A. (eds) (1990) *Postmodernism and Society*, London: Macmillan.

Bozalek, V. (1999) Unpublished part of published paper 'Feminist Postmodernism in the South African Context' in Fawcett, B., Featherstone, B., Fook, J. and Rossiter, A. (eds) *Researching and Practising in Social Work: Postmodern Feminist Perspectives*, London: Routledge.

Brah, A. (1992) 'Difference, Diversity and Differentiation' in Donald, J. and Rattansi, A. (eds) *'Race', Culture and Difference*, London: Sage/ Open University Press, pp. 126–45.

Braye, S. and Preston-Shoot, M. (1995) *Empowering Practice in Social Care*, Buckingham: Open University Press.

Briskin, L. (1990) 'Identity Politics and the Hierarchy of Oppression: A Comment' in *Feminist Review* **34–36**: 102–8.

Brodrib, S. (1992) *Nothing Mat(t)ers: A Feminist Critique of Postmodernism*, Melbourne: Spinnifex.

Broverman, D., Clarkson, F., Rosenkrantz, P., Vogel, S. and Broverman, I. (1970) 'Sex-role Stereotype and Clinical Judgements of Mental Health' in *Journal of Consulting and Clinical Psychiatry*, **34**: 1–7.

Bryant, C. and Jary, D. (eds) (1991) *Giddens' Theory of Structuration: A Critical Appreciation*, London: Routledge.

Burr, V. (1995) *An Introduction to Social Constructionism*, London: Routledge.

Bury, M. (1996) 'Defining and Researching Disability: Challenges and Responses' in Barnes, C. and Mercer, G. (eds) *Exploring the Divided: Illness and Disability*, Leeds: The Disability Press, pp. 17–38.

Busfield, J. (1996) *Men, Women, and Madness: Understanding Gender and Mental Disorder,* Basingstoke: Macmillan.

Butler, J. (1990) *Gender Trouble: Feminism and the Subversion of Identity,* London: Routledge.

Butler, J. (1993) *Bodies That Matter: On the Discursive Limits of 'Sex',* London: Routledge.

Butler, J. (1995) 'Contingent Foundations: Feminism and the Question of Postmodernism' in Nicholson, L. (ed.) *Feminist Contentions: A Philosophical Exchange,* London: Routledge, pp. 35–57.

Bynoe, I., Oliver, M. and Barnes, C. (1991) *Equal Rights for Disabled People: The Case for a New Law,* London: IPPR.

Cahoone, L. (1996) 'Introduction' in Cahoone, L. (ed.) *From Modernism to Postmodernism: An Anthology,* Oxford: Blackwell.

Cain, M. (1993) 'Foucault, Feminism and Feeling – What Foucault Can and Cannot Contribute to Feminist Epistemology' in Ramazanoğlu, C. (ed.) *Up Against Foucault: Explorations of Some Tensions Between Foucault and Feminism,* London: Routledge, pp. 73–96.

Carby, H. (1982) 'Black Feminism and the Boundaries of Sisterhood' in *The Empire Strikes Back: 'Race' and Racism in 70's Britain,* London: Hutchinson.

Challis, D. (1994) 'Case Management: A Review of UK Developments and Issues' in Titterton, M. (ed.) *Caring for People in the Community,* London: Jessica Kingsley, pp. 91–112.

Challis, D., Chessum, R., Chesterman, J., Luckett, R. and Traske, K. (1990) *Case Management in Social and Health Care,* Canterbury: Personal Social Services Research Unit.

Chodorow, N. J. (1994) *Femininities, Masculinities, Sexualities: Freud and Beyond,* London: Free Association Books.

Christian, B. (1988) 'The Race for Theory' in *Feminist Studies,* **14**: 67–9.

Cixous, H. (1994) in Sellers, S. (ed.) *The Helene Cixous Reader,* London: Routledge.

Clarke, J. (1996) 'After Social Work?' in Parton, N. (ed.) *Social Theory, Social Change and Social Work,* London: Routledge, pp. 36–60.

Clegg, S. R. (1992) *Frameworks of Power,* London: Sage.

Coleridge, P. (1993) *Disability, Liberation and Development,* Oxford: Oxfam.

Community Care Magazine (1999) 'Survey of Social Workers' Attitudes to Management' in *Community Care Magazine,* 6–12 May 1999.

Connell, R. W. (1985) 'Theorising Gender' in *Sociology,* **19**(2): 260–72.

Connolly, C. (1990) 'Splintered Sisterhood: Anti-Racism in a Young Women's Project' in *Feminist Review,* **36**: 52–64.

Corker, M. and French, S. (eds) (1999) *Disability Discourse,* Buckingham: Open University Press.

Cotterill, P. (1992) 'Interviewing Women: Issues of Friendship, Vulnerability and Power' in *Women's Studies International Forum*, 15(5–6): 593–606.

Croft, S. and Beresford, P. (1992) *Involving People in Social Services: From Paternalism to Participation*, London: Open Service Project/Joseph Rowntree Foundation.

Crow, L. (1996) 'Including All of Our Lives: Renewing the Social Model of Disability' in Barnes, C. and Mercer, G. (eds) *Exploring the Divide: Illness and Disability*, Leeds: The Disability Press, pp. 55–73.

CSO (1998) *Social Trends*, London: HMSO.

Cumberbatch, G. and Negrie, R. (1992) *Images of Disability on Television*, London: Routledge.

Dalley, G. (1988) *Ideologies of Caring: Rethinking Community and Collectivism*, London: Macmillan.

Dalley, G. (1993) 'The Principles of Collective Care' in Bornat, J., Pereira, C., Pilgrim, D. and Williams, F. (eds) *Community Care: A Reader*, Basingstoke: Macmillan, pp. 152–5.

Davies, A. (1999) 'A Missed Opportunity' in *Community Care Magazine*, 18–24 March 1999, p. 23.

Davies, K., Dickey, J. and Stratford, T. (1987) *Out of Focus*, London: Women's Press.

Deleuze, G. and Guattari, F. (1988) *A Thousand Plateaus*, London: Athlone.

Department of Health (1970) *The Chronically Sick and Disabled Persons Act 1970*, London: HMSO.

Department of Health (1986) *The Disabled People (Services Consultation and Representation) Act 1986*, London: HMSO.

Department of Health (1989) *Caring for People: Community Care in the Next Decade and Beyond*, London Cm 849 (White Paper), London: HMSO.

Department of Health (1990a) *Community Care: A Policy Guide for Managers*, London: HMSO.

Department of Health (1990b) *The National Health Service and Community Care Act 1990*, London: HMSO.

Department of Health (1995a) *The Carers (Recognition and Services) Act 1995*, London: HMSO.

Department of Health (1995b) *The Disability Discrimination Act 1995*, London: HMSO.

Department of Health (1995c) *Community Care Development Programme Consultation Document*, London: HMSO.

Department of Health (1996) *The Direct Payments Act 1996*, London: HMSO.

Department of Health (1998a) *Modernising Social Services*, London: HMSO.

Department of Health (1998b) *Welfare Reform Bill*, London: HMSO.

Department of Health (1998c) *Modern Local Government: In Touch with the People*, London: HMSO.

Department of Health and Social Security (1988) *The Griffiths Report: Community Care: Agenda for Action*, London: HMSO.

Department of Health/Social Services Inspectorate (1991) *Training for Community Care: A Joint Approach*, London: HMSO.

Derrida, J. (1978) *Writing and Difference*, trans. A. Bass, Chicago: University of Chicago Press.

Deveaux, M. (1994) 'Feminism and Empowerment: A Critical Reading of Foucault' in *Feminist Studies*, **20**(2) (Summer): 223–47.

Dews, P. (1979) 'The Nouvelle Philosophie and Foucault' in *Economy and Society*, **8**(2): 127–71.

Dickens, D. R. and Fontana, A. (1994) *Postmodernism and Social Inquiry*, London: UCL Press.

Di Stefano, C. (1990) 'Dilemmas of Difference' in Nicholson, L. J. (ed.) *Feminism/Postmodernism*, London: Routledge, pp. 63–82.

Docherty, M. (ed.) (1993) *Postmodernism: A Reader*, Hemel Hempstead: Harvester Wheatsheaf.

Donald, J. and Rattansi, A. (eds) (1992) *'Race', Culture and Difference*, London: Open University Press/Sage.

Douglas, M. (1966) *Purity and Danger*, Harmondsworth: Penguin.

Dowson, S. (1990) *Keeping it Safe: Self Advocacy of People with Learning Difficulty and the Professional Response*, London: Values Into Action.

Doyal, L. and Gough, I. (1991) *A Theory of Human Need*, Basingstoke: Macmillan.

Drake, R. F. (1999) *Understanding Disability Policies*, Macmillan: Basingstoke.

Dreyfus, H. L. and Rabinow, P. (eds) (1993) *Michel Foucault: Beyond Structuralism and Hermeneutics*, Chicago: University of Chicago Press.

Driedger, D. (1989) *The Last Civil Rights Movement*, London: Hurst and Company.

Edley, N. and Wetherell, M. (1997) 'Jockeying for Position: On the Construction of Masculine Identities' in *Discourse and Society*, London: Sage, pp. 203–15.

Edwards, D. (1996) *Discourse and Cognition*, London: Sage.

Edwards, T. (1994) *Erotics and Politics: Gay Male Sexuality, Masculinity and Feminism*, London: Routledge.

Eisenstein, H. (1984) *Contemporary Feminist Thought*, London: Allen and Unwin.

Faith, K. (1994) 'Resistance: Lessons from Foucault and Feminism' in Radtke, H. L. and Stam, H. J. (eds) *Power/Gender Social Relations in Theory and Practice*, London: Sage, pp. 36–66.

Fawcett, B. (1996a) 'Postmodernism, Feminism and Disability' in *Scandinavian Journal of Social Welfare*, **1996**(5): 259–67.

Fawcett, B. (1996b) 'Women, Mental Health and Community Care: An Abusive Combination?' in Fawcett, B., Featherstone, B., Hearn, J. and Toft, C. (eds) *Violence and Gender Relations: Theories and Interventions*, London: Sage, pp. 81–97.

Fawcett, B. (1998) 'Disability and Social Work: Applications from Poststructuralism, Postmodernism and Feminism' in *British Journal of Social Work*, **28**: 263–77.

Fawcett, B. (1999a) 'Researching Disability: Meanings, Interpretation and Analysis' in Fawcett, B., Featherstone, B., Fook, J. and Rossiter, A. (eds) *Researching and Practising in Social Work: Postmodern Feminist Perspectives*, London: Routledge.

Fawcett, B. (1999b) *Theorising Postmodern Feminism and Disability: A Qualitative and Deconstructive Study of Disability Amongst Disabled People*, PhD Thesis, Manchester, Manchester University.

Fawcett, B. and Featherstone, B. (1994a) 'Power and Difference: Perspectives for Practice' in Fawcett, B., Featherstone, B. and Toft, C. (eds) *Women, the System and Mental Health*, Bradford: Bradford University Publication, pp. 41–7.

Fawcett, B. and Featherstone, B. (1994b) 'The Implications of Community Care Policies for People who Require and Use Services' in *Care in Place: The International Journal of Networks and Community*, **1**(2): 120–32.

Fawcett, B. and Featherstone, B. (1996) ' "Carers" and "Caring": New Thoughts on Old Questions' in Humphries, B. (ed.) *Critical Perspectives on Empowerment*, Birmingham: Venture Press, pp. 53–68.

Fawcett, B. and Featherstone, B. (1998) 'Quality Assurance and Evaluation in Social Work in a Postmodern Era' in Carter, J. (ed.) *Postmodernity and the Fragmentation of Welfare*, London: Routledge, pp. 67–82.

Fawcett, B. and Featherstone, B. (1999) 'Setting the Scene: An Appraisal of Notions of Postmodernism, Postmodernity and Postmodern Feminism' in Fawcett, B., Featherstone, B., Fook, J. and Rossiter, A. (eds) *Researching and Practising in Social Work: Postmodern Feminist Perspectives*, London: Routledge.

Featherstone, B. and Fawcett, B. (1995) 'Oh No! Not More Isms: Feminism, Postmodernism and Poststructuralism and Social Work Education' in *Social Work Education*, **14**(3) (Autumn): 25–43.

Fine, M. and Asch, A. (eds) (1988) *Women with Disabilities: Essays in Psychology, Culture and Politics*, Philadelphia: Temple University Press.

Finkelstein, V. (1993a) 'The Commonality of Disability' in Swain, J., Finkelstein, V., French, S. and Oliver, M. (eds) *Disabling Barriers – Enabling Environments*, London: Sage, pp. 9–16.

Finkelstein, V. (1993b) 'Disability: An Administrative Challenge? (The Health and Welfare Heritage)' in Oliver, M. (ed.) *Social Work: Disabled People and Disabling Environments, Research Highlights in Social Work 2*, London: Jessica Kingsley, pp. 19–39.

Fisher, M. (1994) 'Man-made Care: Community Care and Older Male Carers' in *British Journal of Social Work*, **24**: 659–80.

Flax, J. (1990) *Thinking Fragments, Psychoanalysis, Feminism and Postmodernism in the Contemporary West*, Berkeley: University of California Press.

Flax, J. (1992a) 'The End of Innocence' in Butler, J. and Scott, J. (eds) *Feminists Theorise the Political*, London: Routledge, pp. 445–63.

Flax, J. (1992b) 'Beyond Equality, Gender, Justice and Difference' in Bock, L. and James, S. (eds) *Beyond Equality and Difference*, London: Routledge, pp. 193–210.

Fook, J. (1999) 'Deconstructing and Reconstructing Professional Expertise' in Fawcett, B., Featherstone, B., Fook, J. and Rossiter, A. (eds) *Researching and Practising in Social Work: Postmodern Feminist Perspectives*, London: Routledge.

Foucault, M. (1972) *The Archaeology of Knowledge*, London: Tavistock.

Foucault, M. (1979) *Discipline and Punish*, Harmondsworth: Penguin.

Foucault, M. (1980) in Gordon, C. (ed.) *Michel Foucault: Power/Knowledge: Selected Interviews and Other Writings 1972–1977 by Michel Foucault*, Hemel Hempstead: Harvester Wheatsheaf.

Foucault, M. (1981a) *The History of Sexuality, Volume One, An Introduction*, Harmondsworth: Pelican.

Foucault, M. (1981b) 'Question of Method: An Interview with Michel Foucault' in *Ideology and Consciousness*, **8**: 1–14.

Foucault, M. (1983) in Dreyfus, H. L. and Rabinow, P. (eds) *Michel Foucault: Beyond Structuralism and Hermeneutics*, Chicago: University of Chicago Press.

Foucault, M. (1986) *The History of Sexuality, Volume Two, The Use of Pleasure*, Harmondsworth: Viking.

Foucault, M. (1991) in Rabinow, P. (ed.) *The Foucault Reader*, Harmondsworth: Penguin.

Fox, N. J. (1991) 'Postmodernism, Rationality and the Evaluation of Health Care' in *Sociological Review*, **39**: 709–44.

Fox, N. J. (1993) *Postmodernism, Sociology and Health*, Buckingham: Open University Press.

Fraser, N. (1993) *Unruly Practices: Power, Discourse and Gender in Contemporary Social Theory*, Cambridge: Polity Press.

Fraser, N. (1995) 'False Antithesis: A Response to Seyla Benhabib and Judith Butler' in Nicholson, L. (ed.) *Feminist Contentions: A Philosophical Exchange*, London: Routledge, pp. 59–74.

Fraser, N. and Nicholson, L. (1993) 'Social Criticism Without Philosophy: An Encounter Between Feminism and Postmodernism' in Docherty, M. (ed.) *Postmodernism: A Reader*, Hemel Hempstead: Harvester Wheatsheaf, pp. 415–32.

French, S. (1993) 'Disability, Impairment or Something in Between' in Swain, J., Finkelstein, V., French, S. and Oliver, M. (eds) *Disabling Barriers – Enabling Environments*, London: Open University Press/Sage, pp. 17–25.

Garland-Thompson, R. G. (1994) 'Re-drawing the Boundaries of Feminist Disability Studies' in *Feminist Studies*, **20**(3): 583–97.

Gerschick, T. J. and Miller, A. S. (1995) 'Coming to Terms: Masculinity and Physical Disability' in Sabo, D. and Gordon, D. F. (eds) *Men's Health and Illness*, Thousand Oaks, CA: Sage, pp. 183–204.

Giddens, A. (1984) *The Constitution of Society*, Cambridge: Polity Press.

Giddens, A. (1990) *The Consequences of Modernity*, Cambridge: Polity Press.

Giddens, A. (1991) *Modernity and Self Identity*, Cambridge: Polity Press.

Gilroy, P. (1992) 'The End of Anti-Racism' in Donald, J. and Rattansi, A. (eds) *'Race', Culture and Difference*, London: Open University Press/Sage, pp. 49–61.

Godfery, M. and Wistow, G. (1997) 'The User Perspective on Managing Health Outcomes: The Case of Mental Health' in *Health and Social Care in the Community*, **5**(5): 325–32.

Gordon, C. (ed.) (1980) *Michel Foucault: Power/Knowledge: Selected Interviews and other Writings 1972–1977 by Michel Foucault*, Hemel Hempstead: Harvester Wheatsheaf.

Gorman, J. (1992) *Out of the Shadows*, London: Mind Publications.

Graham, H. (1994) *Women, Health and the Family*, Brighton: Wheatsheaf.

Graham, H. (1997) 'Feminist Perspectives on Caring' in Bornat, J., Johnson, J., Pereira, C., Pilgrim, D. and Williams, F. (eds) *Community Care: A Reader*, second edition, Basingstoke: Open University Press/Macmillan, pp. 124–33.

Green, D. G. (1996) *Community Without Politics: A Market Approach to Welfare Reform*, London: IEA Health and Welfare Unit, Choice in Welfare, No. 27.

Green, H. (1988) *Informal Carers*, London: General Household Survey, HMSO.

Grosz, E. (1987) 'Feminist Theory and the Challenge to Knowledges' in *Women's Studies International Forum*, **10**(5): 475–80.

Grosz, E. (1994) *Volatile Bodies: Towards a Corporeal Feminism*, Bloomington and Indianapolis: Indiana University Press.

Habermas, J. (1981) 'Modernity versus Postmodernity' in *New German Critique*, **22**: 3–14.

Hacking, I. (1986) 'Making Up People' in Helier, T. C. (ed.) *Reconstructing Individualism*, Stanford: Stanford University Press.

Hahn H. (1988) 'Can Disability be Beautiful' in *Social Policy*, **18** (Winter): 26–31.

Halberg, M. (1989) 'Feminist Epistemology: An Impossible Project?' in *Radical Philosophy*, **53** (Autumn): 3–6.

Hales, G. (ed.) (1996) *Beyond Disability: Towards an Enabling Society*, London: Sage/Open University Press.

Hanmer, J. and Saunders, S. (1984) *Well Founded Fear: A Community Study of Violence to Women*, London: Hutchinson.

Hanmer, J. and Statham, D. (1992) *Women and Social Work: Towards a Woman-Centred Practice*, Basingstoke: BASW/Macmillan.

Harding, S. (1986) *The Science in Question*, Ithaca, NY: Cornell University Press.

Harding, S. (1990) 'Feminism, Science and the Anti-Enlightenment Critique' in Nicholson, L. (ed.) *Feminism/Postmodernism*, London: Routledge, pp. 83–106.

Harper, D. (1995) 'Discourse Analysis and Mental Health' in *Journal of Mental Health*, **4**: 347–57.

Harris, A., Cox, E. and Smith, C. (1971) *Handicapped and Impaired in Great Britain, Economic Dimensions*, London: HMSO.

Hartsock, N. (1990) 'Foucault on Power: A Theory for Women' in Nicholson, L. (ed.) *Feminism/Postmodernism*, London: Routledge, pp. 157–75.

Hartsock, N. (1996) 'Postmodernism and Political Change: Issues for Feminist Theory' in Hekman, S. J. (ed.) *Feminist Interpretations of Michel Foucault*, Pennsylvania: Pennsylvania State University Press.

Harvey, D. (1989) *The Condition of Postmodernity*, London: Blackwell.

Harvey, L. (1992) *Critical Social Research*, London: Unwin Hyman.

Healy, K. and Peile, C. (1995) 'From Silence to Activism: Approaches to Research and Practice with Young Mothers' in *Affilia*, **10**(3): 280–98.

Hearn, J. (1992) *Men in the Public Eye*, London: Routledge.

Hearn, J. (1994) 'The Organisation(s) of Violence: Men, Gender Relations, Organisations and Violences' in *Human Relations*, **47**(6): 1–23.

Hearn, J. (1996) 'Men's Violence to Known Women: Historical, Everyday and Theoretical Constructions by Men' in Fawcett, B., Featherstone, B., Hearn, J. and Toft, C. (eds) *Violence and Gender Relations: Theories and Interventions*, London: Sage, pp. 22–37.

Hearn, J. (1998) 'Theorising Men and Men's Theorising: Varieties of Discursive Practices in Men's Theorising of Men' in *Theory and Society*, **27**(6): 781–816.

Hearn, J. and Morgan, D. H. J. (1995) 'Contested Discourses on Men and Masculinities' in Blair, M. and Holland, J. with Sheldon, S. (eds) *Identity and Diversity: Gender and the Experience of Education*, Clevedon: Multilingual Matters in association with the Open University Press, pp. 173–85.

Hearn, J. and Parkin, W. (1993) 'Organisation, Multiple Oppressions and Postmodernism' in Parker, M. and Hassard, J. (eds) *Postmodernism and Organisation Theory*, London: Sage, pp. 148–62.

Hearn, J., Sheppard, D. L., Tancred-Sheriff, P. and Burrell, G. (eds) (1989) *The Sexuality of Organisation*, London: Sage.

Hekman, S. (1990) *Gender and Knowledge: Elements of a Postmodern Feminism*, Cambridge: Polity Press.

Hekman, S. (1995) *Moral Voices, Moral Selves: Carol Gilligan and Feminist Moral Theory*, Cambridge: Polity Press.

Hevey, D. (1992) *The Creatures Time Forgot*, London: Routledge.

Heyman, B. (ed.) (1998) *Risks, Health and Health Care*, London: Arnold.

Heyman, B. and Henrikson, M. (1998a) 'Values and Health Risks' in Heyman, B. (ed.) *Risk, Health and Health Care*, London: Arnold.

Heyman, B. and Henrikson, M. (1998b) 'Probability and Health Risks' in Heyman, B. (ed.) *Risk, Health and Health Care*, London: Arnold, pp. 27–64.

Hill Collins, P. (1989) 'The Social Construction of Black Feminist Thought' in *Signs: Journal of Women in Culture and Society*, **14**(4): 745–73.

Hill Collins, P. (1991) *Black Feminist Thought*, New York: Routledge.

Hirst, P. (1994) *Associative Democracy: New Forums of Economic and Social Governance*, Cambridge: Polity Press, pp. 65–105.

Hollway, W. (1989) *Subjectivity and Method in Psychology: Gender, Meaning and Science*, London: Sage.

Hollway, W. (1996) 'Gender and Power in Organizations' in Fawcett, B., Featherstone, B., Hearn, J. and Toft, C. (eds) *Violence and Gender Relations: Theories and Interventions*, London: Sage, pp. 72–80.

hooks, B. (1991) *Yearning: Race and Gender and Cultural Politics*, London: Turnaround Press.

Howe, D. (1994) 'Modernity, Postmodernity and Social Work' in *British Journal of Social Work*, **24**: 513–32.

Howe, D. (1996) 'Surface and Depth in Social Work Practice' in Parton, N. (ed.) *Social Theory, Social Change and Social Work*, London: Routledge, pp. 77–97.

Hugman, R. and Smith, D. (eds) (1995) *Ethical Issues in Social Work*, London: Routledge.

Humphries, B. (ed.) (1996) *Critical Perspectives on Empowerment*, Birmingham: Venture Press.

Hurst, J. (1999) 'Is This a Land Fit for Unsung Heroes' in *Community Care Magazine*, 18–24 February 1999, pp. 8–9.

Huyssen, A. (1990) 'Mapping the Postmodern' in Nicholson, L. (ed.) *Feminism/Postmodernism*, London: Routledge, pp. 234–77.

Irigaray, L. (1993) *Je, Tu, Nous: Towards a Culture of Difference*, trans. A. Martin, London: Routledge.

Jackson, S. (1992) 'The Amazing Deconstructing Woman' in *Trouble and Strife*, **25**: 25–31.

Jackson, S. (1993) *Women's Studies: A Reader*, Hemel Hempstead: Harvester Wheatsheaf.

James, S. M. (1993) 'Introduction' in James, S. M. and Busia, P. A. (eds) *Theorising Black Feminisms*, London: Routledge.

Jameson, F. (1993) 'Postmodernism or the Cultural Logic of Late Capitalism' in Docherty, T. (ed.) *Postmodernisms: A Reader*, Hemel Hempstead: Harvester Wheatsheaf, pp. 62–92.

Jary, D. and Jary, J. (1991) *The Collins Dictionary of Sociology*, Glasgow: Harper Collins.

Jenness, V. (1992) 'Coming Out: Lesbian Identities and the Categorization Problem' in Plummer, K. (ed.) *Modern Homosexualities*, London: Routledge, pp. 65–74.

Johnston, M. (1997) 'Integrating Models of Disability: A Reply to Shakespcare and Watson' in Barton, L. and Oliver, M. (eds) *Disability Studies: Past, Present and Future*, Leeds: The Disability Press, pp. 281–5.

Jones, K., Brown, J. and Bradshaw, J. (1978) *Issues in Social Policy*, London: Routledge and Kegan Paul.

Jones, L. I. (1994) *The Social Context of Health and Welfare*, Macmillan: Basingstoke.

Kelly, L., Burton, S. and Regan, L. (1994) 'Researching Women's Lives or Studying Women's Oppression? Reflections on What Constitutes Feminist Research' in Maynard, M. and Purvis, J. (eds) *Researching Women's Lives from a Feminist Perspective*, London: Taylor and Francis, pp. 27–48.

Kestenbaum, A. with Cava, H. (1998) *Work, Rest and Pay: The Deal for Personal Assistance Users*, York: J. R. Foundation.

Kristeva, J. (1986) *The Kristeva Reader*, Oxford: Blackwell.

Langan, M. and Day, L. (eds) (1992) *Women, Oppression and Social Work*, London: Routledge.

Law Commission (1995) *Mental Incapacity*, London: HMSO.

Layder, D. (1994) *Understanding Social Theory*, London: Sage.

Leder, D. (1990) *The Absent Body*, Chicago: University of Chicago Press.

Lenny, J. (1993) 'Do Disabled People Need Counselling' in Swain, J., Finkelstein, V., French, S. and Oliver, M. (eds) *Disabling Barriers*

– *Enabling Environments*, London: Open University Press/Sage, pp. 233–40.

Levi-Strauss, C. (1949) *The Elementary Structures of Kinship*, Boston: Beacon Press.

Lewis, J. and Glennerster, H. (1996) *Implementing the New Community Care*, Buckingham: Open University Press.

LGMP (1998) London: Local Government Management Publications.

Liberty (1994) *Women's Rights, Human Rights*, London: National Council for Civil Liberties.

Lister, R. (1993) Book Review of 'Disability, Citizenship and Empowerment', K665 The Disabling Society Workbook 2, M. Oliver 1993 in *Disability, Handicap and Society*, **8**(3): 329–34.

Lister, R. (1997) *Citizenship: Feminist Perspectives*, Basingstoke: Macmillan.

Lister, R. (1998) 'Citizenship and Difference: Towards a Differentiated Universalism' in *European Journal of Social Theory*, **1**(1) (July): 71–90.

Lloyd, M. (1995) 'Does She Boil Eggs? Towards a Feminist Model of Disability' in Blair, M. and Holland, J. with Sheldon, S. (eds) *Identity and Diversity: Gender and the Experience of Education*, Clevedon: Multilingual Matters in association with the Open University Press, pp. 211–24.

Longmore, P. K. (1987) 'Screening Stereotypes, Images of Disabled People in Television and Motion Pictures' in Gartner, A. and Joe, T. (eds) *Images of the Disabled, Disabling Images*, New York: Praeger.

Lonsdale, S. (1990) *Women and Disability: The Experience of Physical Disability Among Women*, Women in Society Series, Basingstoke: Macmillan.

Lorde, A. (1984) *Sister Outsider*, California: Crossing Press Feminist Series.

Lovibond, S. (1993) 'Feminism and Postmodernism' in Docherty, T. (ed.) *Postmodernism: A Reader*, Hemel Hempstead: Harvester Wheatsheaf, pp. 390–414.

Lukes, S. (1974) *Power: A Radical View*, London: Macmillan.

Lupton, D. (1997) 'Doctors and the Medical Profession' in *Sociology of Health and Illness*, **19**(4): 480–97.

Lyotard, J. F. (1984) *The Postmodern Condition: A Report on Knowledge*, Manchester: Manchester University Press.

Lyotard, J. F. (1988) *The Differend: Phases in Dispute*, Manchester: Manchester University Press.

Macdonell, D. (1986) *Theories of Discourse: An Introduction*, Oxford: Blackwell.

Mandelstam, M. with Schwehr, B. (1996) *Community Care Practice and the Law*, London and Bristol: Jessica Kingsley.

Manthorpe, J., Walsh, M. with Alaszewski, A. and Harrison, L. (1997) 'Issues of Risk, Practice and Welfare in Learning Disability Services' in *Disability and Society*, **12**(1): 69–82.

Marshall, T. H. (1952) *Citizenship and Social Class*, Cambridge: Cambridge University Press.

Maynard, M. (1994) 'Methods, Practice and Epistemology: The Debate about Feminism and Research' in Maynard, M. and Purvis, J. (eds) *Researching Women's Lives from a Feminist Perspective*, London: Taylor and Francis, pp. 10–26.

Mayo, M. (1994) *Communities and Caring: The Mixed Economy of Welfare*, Basingstoke: Macmillan.

McBeath, G. B. and Webb, S. A. (1991) 'Social Work, Modernity and Postmodernity' in *Sociological Review*, **39**(4): 755–62.

McDowell, L. and Pringle, R. (eds) *Defining Women: Social Institutions and Gender Divisions*, Cambridge: Polity Press/Open University Press.

McKee, A. (1982) 'The Feminisation of Poverty' in *Graduate Woman*, **76**(4): 34–6.

McNay, L. (1992) *Foucault and Feminism*, Oxford: Blackwell.

McNay, M. (1992) 'Social Work and Power Relations: Towards a Framework for an Integrated Practice' in Langan, M. and Day, L. (eds) *Women, Oppression and Social Work*, London: Routledge, pp. 48–66.

McNeil, M. (1993) 'Dancing with Foucault' in Ramazanoğlu, C. (ed.) *Up Against Foucault: Explorations of Some Tensions Between Foucault and Feminism*, London: Routledge.

Means, R. and Smith, R. (1998) *Community Care: Policy and Practice*, revised edition, Basingstoke: Macmillan.

Meredith, B. (1995) *The Community Care Handbook: The Reformed System Explained*, London: Age Concern.

Merquior, J. G. (1985) *Foucault*, London: Fontana.

Moore, H. L. (1994) *A Passion for Difference*, Cambridge: Polity Press.

Moore, M., Beazley, S. and Maelzer, J. (1998) *Researching Disability*, Buckingham: Open University Press.

Morris, J. (1991) ' "Us" and "Them"? Feminist Research, Community Care and Disability' in *Critical Social Policy*, **31–33**: 22–39.

Morris, J. (1993a) *Pride Against Prejudice*, London: Women's Press.

Morris, J. (1993b) *Independent Lives: Community Care and Disabled People*, Basingstoke: Macmillan.

Morris, J. (1996a) *Encounters with Strangers: Feminism and Disability*, London: Women's Press.

Morris, J. (1996b) *Encouraging User Involvement in Commissioning: A Resource for Commissioners*, London: Department of Health.

Morris, M. (1988) *The Pirates Fiancee: Feminism, Reading Postmodernism,* London: Verso.

Nicholson, J. (1993) *Postmodernism, Sociology and Health,* Buckingham: Open University Press.

Nicholson, L. (ed.) (1990) *Feminism/Postmodernism,* London: Routledge.

Nicholson, L. (ed.) (1995) *Feminist Contentions: A Philosophical Exchange,* London: Routledge.

Nicholson, L. and Seidman, S. (eds) (1995) *Social Postmodernism: Beyond Identity Politics,* Cambridge: Cambridge University Press.

Nuffield Institute for Health/Kings Fund (1998) *Our Turn Next,* Leeds: The Nuffield Institute.

Office of Population Censuses and Surveys, *Handicapped and Impaired in Great Britain,* London: HMSO.

Oliver, M. (1983) *Social Work with Disabled People,* Basingstoke: Macmillan.

Oliver, M. (1990) *The Politics of Disablement,* Basingstoke: Macmillan.

Oliver, M. (1992) *Social Work with Disabled People,* Basingstoke: BASW/ Macmillan.

Oliver, M. (ed.) (1993) *Social Work: Disabled People and Disabling Environments, Research Highlights in Social Work 2,* London: Jessica Kingsley.

Oliver, M. (1996) *Understanding Disability: From Theory to Practice,* Basingstoke: Macmillan.

Oliver, M. and Barnes, C. (1998) *Disabled People and Social Policy: From Exclusion to Inclusion,* London: Longman.

OPCS (Office of Population Censuses and Surveys) (1971) *Handicapped and Impaired in Britain,* London: HMSO.

Open University (1993) 'Meanings and Perspectives in Community Care' in *Community Care Workbook 1,* K259 WB1, Milton Keynes: Open University.

Opie, A. (1990) 'Caring for the Confused Elderly at Home' in *New Zealand Women's Studies Journal,* **6**(1–2): 46–64.

Opie, A. (1992) 'Qualitative Research, Appropriation of the "Other" and Empowerment' in *Feminist Review,* **40–42**: 52–69.

Orme, J. (1998) 'Community Care: Gender Issues in Critical Commentaries' in *British Journal of Social Work,* **28**: 615–22.

Palmer, P. (1989) *Contemporary Women's Fiction,* London: Harvester.

Parsons T. (1951) *The Social System,* London: Routledge and Kegan Paul.

Parton, N. (1994) 'Problematics of Government (Post) Modernity and Social Work' in *British Journal of Social Work,* **24**(1): 9–32.

Payne, M. (1991) *Modern Social Work Theory,* Basingstoke: Macmillan.

Payne, M. (1995) *Social Work and Community Care*, Basingstoke: Macmillan.

Pease, B. (1999) 'Researching Men's Narratives: Participatory Methodologies in a Postmodern Frame' in Fawcett, B., Featherstone, B., Fook, J. and Rossiter, A. (eds) *Researching and Practising in Social Work: Postmodern Feminist Perspectives*, London: Routledge.

Pereira, C. (1997) 'Introduction' in Bornat, J., Johnson, J., Pereira, C., Pilgrim, D. and Williams, F. (eds) *Community Care: A Reader*, second edition, Basingstoke: Open University Press/Macmillan, pp. xi–xii.

Philp, M. (1979) 'Notes on the Form of Knowledge in Social Work' in *Sociological Review*, **21**(1): 83–111.

Pinder, R. (1995) 'Bringing Back the Body Without the Blame? The Experience of Ill and Disabled People at Work' in *Sociology of Health and Illness*, **17**: 605–31.

Pinder, R. (1996) 'Sick-but-Fit or Fit-but-Sick? Ambiguity and Identity at the Workplace' in Barnes, C. and Mercer, G. (eds) *Exploring the Divide: Illness and Disability*, Leeds: The Disability Press, pp. 135–56.

Pinder, R. (1997) 'A Reply to Tom Shakespeare and Nicholas Watson' in Barton, L. and Oliver, M. (eds) *Disability Studies: Past, Present and Future*, Leeds: The Disability Press, pp. 274–80.

Plummer, K. (1995) *Telling Sexual Stories*, London: Routledge.

Pozatek, E. (1994) 'The Problem of Certainty: Clinical Social Work in the Postmodern Era' in *Social Work*, **39**(4): 396–402.

Price, J. (1996) 'The Marginal Politics of Our Bodies? Women's Health, The Disability Movement and Power' in Humphries, B. (ed.) *Critical Perspectives on Empowerment*, Birmingham: Venture Press, pp. 35–52.

Prince, J. (1993) 'Introduction to Women, Education and Work' in Jackson, S. (ed.) *Women's Studies: A Reader*, London: Harvester Wheatsheaf, pp. 133–6.

Rabinow, P. (ed.) (1991) *The Foucault Reader*, Harmondsworth: Penguin.

Radtke, H. L. and Stam, H. J. (eds) (1994) *Power/Gender: Social Relations in Theory and Practice*, London: Sage.

Ramazanoğlu, C. (ed.) (1993) *Up Against Foucault: Explorations of Some Tensions Between Foucault and Feminism*, London: Routledge.

Rattansi, A. (1995) 'Just Framing: Ethnicities and Racisms in a "Postmodern" Framework' in Nicholson, L. and Seidman, S. (eds) *Social Postmodernism: Beyond Identity Politics*, Cambridge: Cambridge University Press, pp. 250–86.

Rose, H. and Bruce, E. (1995) 'Mutual Care But Differential Esteem: Caring Between Older Couples' in Arber, S. and Ginn, J. (eds) *Connecting Gender and Ageing: A Sociological Approach*, Buckingham: Open University Press, pp. 114–28.

Rossiter, A., Prilleltensky, I. and Walsh-Bowers, R. (1999) 'A Postmodern Perspective on Professional Ethics' in Fawcett, B.,

Featherstone, B., Fook, J. and Rossiter, A. (eds) *Researching and Practising in Social Work: Postmodern Feminist Perspectives*, London: Routledge.

Said, E. (1978) *Orientalism*, London: Penguin.

Sands, R. and Nuccio, K. (1992) 'Postmodern Feminist Theory and Social Work' in *Social Work*, **7**(6): 482–94.

Sarup, M. (1993) *Poststructuralism and Postmodernism*, Hemel Hempstead: Harvester Wheatsheaf.

Saussure, F. de (1974) *Course in General Linguistics*, London: Fontana.

Sawicki, J. (1991) *Disciplining Foucault: Feminism, Power and the Body*, London: Routledge.

Scott, J. W. (1994) 'Deconstructing Equality-versus-Difference: or the Uses of Poststructuralist Theory for Feminism' in McDowell, L. and Pringle, R. (eds) *Defining Women: Social Institutions and Gender Divisions*, Cambridge: Polity Press/Open University Press, pp. 253–64.

Scott, J. (1995) *Sociological Theory: Contemporary Debates*, Aldershot: Edward Elgar.

Scull, A. (1979) *Museums of Madness*, Harmondsworth: Penguin.

Segal, L. (1987) *Is the Future Female? Troubled Thoughts on Contemporary Feminism*, London: Virago.

Seidman, S. (ed.) (1994) *The Postmodern Turn: New Perspectives on Social Theory*, Cambridge: Cambridge University Press.

Sellers, S. (ed.) (1994) *Helene Cixous Reader*, London: Routledge.

Shakespeare, T. (1994) 'Cultural Representation of Disabled People: Dustbins for Disavowal?' in *Disability and Society*, **9**(3): 283–99.

Shakespeare, T. (1996) 'Disability, Identity, Difference' in Barnes, C. and Mercer, G. (eds) *Exploring the Divide: Illness and Disability*, Leeds: The Disability Press, pp. 94–113.

Shakespeare, T. (1999) 'When is a Man Not a Man? When He is Disabled' in Wild, J. (ed.) *Working With Men for Change*, London: UCL Press, pp. 47–58.

Shakespeare, T. and Watson, N. (1997) 'Defending the Social Model' in Barton, L. and Oliver, M. (eds) *Disability Studies: Past, Present and Future*, Leeds: The Disability Press, pp. 263–73.

Shakespeare, W. (1970) *The Tempest*, London and Glasgow: Collins.

Shearer, A. (1981) *Disability, Whose Handicap?* Oxford: Blackwell.

Sheppard, M. (1995) *Care Management and the New Social Work: A Critical Analysis*, London: Whiting and Birch.

Silvers, A. (1994) 'Defective Agents: Equality, Difference and the Tyranny of the Normal' in *Journal of Social Philosophy*, **25** (June): 154–75.

Silvers, A. (1995) 'Reconciling Equality to Difference: Caring (f)or Justice for People with Disabilities' in *Hypatia: A Journal of Feminist Philosophy*, **10**(1): 30–55.

Singh, G. (1992) *'Race' and Social Work From 'Black Pathology' to Black Perspectives*, Bradford: Bradford and Ilkley Community College Race Relations Unit.

Smart, B. (1993) *Postmodernity*, London: Routledge.

Smart, C. (1992) 'Feminist Approaches to Criminology or Postmodern Woman Meets Atavistic Man' in Gelsthorpe, L. and Morris, A. (eds) *Feminist Perspectives in Criminology*, Milton Keynes: Open University Press.

Social Services Inspectorate (1995) *Community Care Development Programme Consultation Document*, London: Department of Health.

Social Services Inspectorate/Audit Commission (1996) *Reviewing Social Services: An Introduction to Joint Reviews of Local Authorities Social Services Functions by the Audit Commission and Social Services Inspectorate*, London: HMSO.

Social Services Inspectorate/Audit Commission (1998) *Getting the Best from Social Services' Second Report*, London: HMSO.

Social Services Inspectorate/National Health Service Monitoring Executive (1994) *Caring for People: Impressions of the First Year*, London: Department of Health.

Social Services Inspectorate/National Health Service Monitoring Executive (1995) *Community Care Monitoring Report: Report of 1994 Self Monitoring National Exercises*, London: Department of Health.

Solomon, B. (1976) *Black Empowerment: Social Work in Oppressed Communities*, New York: Columbia University Press.

Spender, D. (1985) *Man Made Language*, second edition, London: Pandora Press.

Stacey, J. (1988) 'Can There Be a Feminist Ethnography' in *Women's Studies International Forum*, **11**(1): 21–7.

Stalker, K. (1998) 'Some Ethical and Methodological Issues in Research with People with Learning Difficulties' in *Disability and Society*, **13**(1): 5–19.

Stanley, L. (1990) *Feminist Praxis*, London: Routledge.

Stanley, L. and Wise, S. (1983) *Breaking Out: Feminist Consciousness and Feminist Research*, London: Routledge and Kegan Paul.

Stanley, L. and Wise, S. (1993) *Breaking Out Again: Feminist Ontology and Epistemology*, second edition, London: Routledge.

Stevens, A. (1991) *Disability Issues: Developing Anti-Discriminatory Practice*, London: Central Council for Education and Training in Social Work, Improving Social Work Training No. 9.

Stone, D. A. (1984) *The Disabled State*, Philadelphia: Temple University Press.

Stuart, O. (1993) 'Double Oppression: An Appropriate Starting Point?' in Swain, J., Finkelstein, V., French, S. and Oliver, M. (eds) *Disabling*

Barriers – Enabling Environments, London: Open University Press/Sage, pp. 93–100.

Swain, J., Finkelstein, V., French, S. and Oliver, M. (eds) (1993) *Disabling Barriers – Enabling Environments*, London: Open University Press/Sage.

Symonds, A. and Kelly, A. (eds) (1998) *The Social Construction of Community Care*, Basingstoke: Macmillan.

Tallack, D. (1995) *Critical Theory: A Reader*, Hemel Hempstead: Harvester Wheatsheaf.

Taylor, D. (1971) *Explanation and Meaning*, Cambridge: Cambridge University Press.

Taylor-Gooby, P. and Lawson, R. (eds) (1993) *Markets and Managers: New Issues in the Delivery of Welfare*, Buckingham: Open University Press.

Tester, S. (1996) *Community Care for Older People: A Comparative Perspective*, Basingstoke: Macmillan.

The Royal Society (1992) *Risk: Analysis, Perception and Management*. Report of a Royal Society Study Group, London: The Royal Society.

Thomas, C. (1999) 'Narrative Identity and the Disabled Self' in Corker, M. and French, S. (eds) *Disability Discourse*, Buckingham: Open University Press.

Thompson, N. (1993) *Anti-Discriminatory Practice*, Macmillan: Basingstoke.

Titterton, M. (1994) *Caring for People in the Community: The New Welfare*, London and Bristol: Jessica Kingsley.

Trevino, L. (1986) 'Ethical Decision Making in Organisations: A Person–Situation Interactionist Model' in *Academy of Management Review*, 11(3): 601–17.

Turner, B. S. (1996) *The Body and Society*, second edition, London: Sage.

UPIAS (1976) *Fundamental Principles of Disability*, London: Union of Physically Impaired Against Segregation.

Venkatesh, B. (1993) 'Setting Out the Issues: An Interview with B. Venkatesh' in Coleridge, P. (ed.) *Disability, Liberation and Development*, Oxford: Oxfam.

Ville, I., Ravaud, J. F., Diard, C. and Paicheler, H. (1994) 'Self-representations and Physical Impairment: A Social Constructionist Approach' in *Sociology of Health and Illness*, 16(3): 301–21.

Walker, A. (1997) 'Community Care Policy: From Consensus to Conflict' in Bornat, J., Johnson, J., Pereira, C., Pilgrim, D. and Williams, F. (eds) *Community Care; A Reader*, second edition, Basingstoke: Macmillan/Open University Press.

Ward, D. and Mullender, A. (1992) 'Empowerment and Oppression: An Indissoluble Pairing for Contemporary Social Work' in *Critical Social Policy*, 32: 21–30.

Webb, R. and Tossell, D. (1999) *Social Issues for Carers*, second edition, London: Arnold.

Weedon, C. (1987) *Feminist Practice and Poststructuralist Theory*, Oxford: Blackwell.

Welfare Reform Bill (1998) London: HMSO.

Wellard, S. (1999) 'Comment' in *Community Care Magazine*, 4–10 March 1999, p. 10.

Wendell, S. (1996) *The Rejected Body: Feminist Philosophical Reflections on Disability*, London: Routledge.

Wetherell, M. and Maybin, J. (1992) 'The Distributed Self' in Stevens, R. (ed.) *Understanding the Self*, London: Sage.

Wetherell, M. and Potter, J. (1992) *Mapping the Language of Racism: Discourse and the Legitimation of Exploitation*, Hemel Hempstead: Harvester Wheatsheaf.

Wetherell, M., Stiven, H. and Potter, J. (1987) 'Unequal Egalitarianism: A Preliminary Study of Discourses Concerning Gender and Employment Opportunities' in *British Journal of Social Psychology*, **26**: 59–71.

White, M. (1999) 'Comment' in *Community Care Magazine*, 25 February–3 March 1999, p. 2.

Williams, F. (1992) 'Somewhere Over the Rainbow: Universality and Diversity in Social Policy' in Manning, N. and Page, R. (eds) *Social Policy Review 4*, London: Social Policy Association, pp. 200–19.

Williams, F. (1994) 'Michele Barrett: From Marxist to Poststructuralist Feminism' in George, V. and Page, R. (eds) *Modern Thinkers on Welfare*, Hemel Hempstead: Harvester Wheatsheaf.

Williams, F. (1996) 'Postmodernism, Feminism and the Question of Difference' in Parton, N. (ed.) *Social Theory, Social Change and Social Work*, London: Routledge, pp. 61–76.

Williams, F. (1997) 'Women and Community' in Bornat, J., Pereira, C., Pilgrim, D. and Williams, F. (eds) *Community Care: A Reader*, second edition, Basingstoke, Macmillan/Open University Press.

Williams, G. (1996) 'Representing Disability: Some Questions of Phenomenology and Politics' in Barnes, C. and Mercer, G. (eds) *Exploring the Divide: Illness and Disability*, Leeds: The Disability Press, pp. 194–212.

Wood, P. (1980) *International Classification of Impairments, Disabilities and Handicaps*, Geneva: World Health Organisation.

Zola, I. K. (1993) 'Self, Identity and the Naming Question: Reflections on the Language of Disability' in *Social Science and Medicine*, **36**: 167–73.

Index

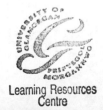